# Terrorism, Mental Health and Aftercare

Roel Van Overmeire

# Terrorism, Mental Health and Aftercare

## A Public Health Perspective

Springer

Roel Van Overmeire
Mental Health and Wellbeing Research Group (MENT)
Vrije Universiteit Brussel
Brussels, Belgium

ISBN 978-3-032-31559-5 ISBN 978-3-032-31560-1 (eBook)
https://doi.org/10.1007/978-3-032-31560-1



This Springer imprint is published by the registered company Springer Nature Switzerland AG
The registered company address is: Gewerbestrasse 11, 6330 Cham, Switzerland

*For Nina.*

# Preface

The term "terrorism" remains alive and kicking in political discourse. Whether it is the 2025 terrorist attacks at Bondi Beach in Australia, or the fear at the time of this writing of future attacks due to the war in Iran, terrorism does not seem alien to the current climate as a word, action, nor fear; one might have expected it to lose importance after the extremist religious wave that spanned several decades, but terrorism remains relevant (though the author is always biased about the importance of this subject).

Yet, despite the title, this book is, in essence, not about terrorism itself, but how it concerns those who are affected by it. It tries to provide an insight into the mental health of the survivors of terrorism: into the psychological and social consequences of experiencing such attacks, as well as all areas of life related to such exposure.

Thus, this book is not just concerned with a psychological look at the subject. In fact, it will say little about the actual "inner mechanisms" of mental health. The reason being that this book has opted for a public health approach, where the discussion of the origin of mental health is secondary to the fact that people can experience mental health issues after terrorist attacks.

Public health, in the author's view, is an approach where one tries to understand and help as much as possible given the limitations of the tools available. Similar to disaster medicine, where one has to make do with the resources available and the situation is anything but ideal for "normal" medicine, so too is it in disaster research that one has to make do with many, many limitations in research, and yet, try to look beyond the limitations for some semblance of data and lessons.

This is therefore also a good place to mention that while percentages of mental health issues are mentioned, they are certainly not the focus of the book. As mentioned, the focus of the book is to provide an understanding of the consequences of terrorism on mental health, and hopefully to provide the reader with general lessons and illustrate them to the reader through many case studies. However, the reader is warned that, as always in social sciences, there are no absolute truths. Context, timing, method, and so many other factors play a role in research.

Additionally, this book is also not meant for just an academic audience. It certainly is written from an academic perspective, but it is also concerned with showing how to improve situations for survivors. Thus, whether the reader is a student, researcher, or, one can hope, a policymaker, this book hopefully provides something for everyone.

The reason for this broader approach is that geopolitical times show the necessity for understanding the consequences of terrorism more. Terrorist attacks have been used as proxies of war—the attacks of ISIS in Europe, while fighting a war in the Levant, are just one of the many, many examples of terrorist attacks being used to affect areas outside the war zone (and as mentioned, the current war in Iran might lead to more such terrorist attacks in other countries). The impact of terrorism is furthermore not just of a humanistic, ethical, research, and health importance, but also of an economic, societal, and policy one. Hence, with regard to policymakers, the lessons in this book on, for example, proactive outreach seem most opportune.

Time also teaches that even if the current geopolitical situation were calm, even then the relevance of this topic would be equally important. After all, on a personal note, while wrapping up my PhD in 2021, I remember ending it with the statement that "the current wave of terrorism" seemed to have ended, and that it might be important to give more attention to the increase of natural disasters due to climate change. Instead, terrorism is at the forefront, together with the threat of war, and "climate", as a word, seems almost taboo. At the time of this writing, the Russian-Ukrainian war is still ongoing and Iran has been bombed by the United States and Israel. One can only hope that a future reader of this book thinks the same as the author at this point in time, namely, that terrorism seems not as relevant as before, though hopefully that will be a more accurate statement at that point in time.

In short, like almost all political scientists, the author is terrible at predicting future political events. Luckily, this is not a political scientific book, nor is it a forward-looking book. It looks back at what we know at this moment of writing.

As it is, the study of how to best help survivors of terrorism is timeless, since even with the best security network, anything can happen. The risk is *never* zero—but it is also never certain that it will happen, one must add.

Content-wise, there are also a few points that need to be mentioned about this book.

**First**, terrorists will not be named, for two reasons. First, terrorism is not the essence of this book; the focus is its consequences. Second, terrorists (at times) seem to strive for fame through violence and destruction. So, while this book is on the effects of terrorism, it should not contribute to a mythologization of the people committing these acts.

**Second**, terminology is important. Throughout the book, post-traumatic stress disorder (PTSD) will be mentioned to refer to all forms of post-traumatic stress studies outcomes. In PTSD studies, often researchers will refer to the outcomes as post-traumatic stress symptoms (PTSS), post-traumatic stress reactions (PTSR), or post-traumatic stress (PTS) (or other variations, for that matter). While PTSD is a controversial term to use in the context of disasters, it seemed more opportune to use PTSD in this context as a "catch-all" term.

Additionally, depression will be used as a term to refer to all studies that have used depression as an outcome, while anxiety is used to refer to all outcomes that measured some form of anxiety. That might seem obvious, but depression can also appear in the form of major depressive disorder (MDD), and anxiety as anxiety disorder.

Related to this, the term "mental health issues" will be mentioned a lot. This is not to dismiss the seriousness of the issues, but to indicate that these are *observational, screened* symptoms, and could be attributed to many things; *they are not by definition evidence of disorders in people.* This also holds true for PTSD, and any other mental health issue mentioned.

Similarly, one of these mental health issues, namely PTSD, is the most mentioned acronym throughout the book. One could certainly argue that this book could have used depression and anxiety outcomes more often, but the majority of studies mentioned in this book used PTSD as an outcome. Considering all of the methodological problems of terrorism studies, differentiating between PTSD, depression, and anxiety for every study that evaluated more than just PTSD, seemed to be inopportune and not useful for the point that is often being made, namely: a rough indication of how many people suffer from mental health issues.

**Third**, what is also important to note is that informed readers might feel certain case studies should have been included in some chapters. For example, Chap. 2 focusses more on 9/11 than on the Oklahoma City Bombing, and does not mention French terrorist attacks often. There are several reasons for this, ranging from the desire to provide more depth to fewer cases, or to provide more diversity (e.g. attacks in India and Japan were included as well). Furthermore, the goal is not to provide the reader with all available research—that is nigh impossible, nor would it be desirable—but to provide the reader insight into, what one can call, the mechanics of mental health problems in the context of terrorist attacks. If experience and knowledge in the field is worth something, the choice of case studies reflects the general principles found across studies, while also providing room for specificities.

**Fourth**, there are no statistical analyses in this book. No doubt there can be a lot of critique to be had on the public health studies, but the priorities differ here from statisticians. While statistics are, at times, a technique for the sake of technique that quite a few people will understand, public health research should lead to the improvement of the health of the public while sometimes, admittedly, quite lacking in technique.

**Fifth**, terrorism studies are a mainly Western field but, all throughout, attempts have been made to provide a global perspective. As such, studies from the United States and France are mentioned alongside studies from Pakistan, Russia, Turkey, and Japan.

And while the geographical width is not as great as that of other disaster fields, this does not take away from the variation in the studies that exist. This book has tried to emulate the richness of the field, while doing justice to the depth of the studies. Hopefully, this goal has been achieved.

This is also a good place to mention that there are quite a lot of terrorist attacks mentioned throughout this book, and the reader can find information on the ones mentioned in this book in the Appendix for reference.

To end this preface, the obvious disclaimer is: even authors of scientific books have certain preferences, and these might come at the cost of aspects that others might feel are more important. By no means is this book the final word on mental health after terrorism. It is simply the word of one researcher in a large room full of voices. It is the cumulation of all I have learned over 8 years, and in any book the author must be arrogant and assume that they know at least *something* interesting about the topic, and with some luck they can even state some form of original insight, without too much obfuscation. Though, despite an author's intent, it is up to the reader to decide if those assumptions hold up.

Brussels, Belgium — Roel Van Overmeire

# Acknowledgements

This first version of this book was finished on 22/03/2026, which is exactly 10 years after the attacks in Belgium; the attacks that were the basis for my PhD and the reason this book exists (or better, the reason why *I* wrote this book). I still remember the interviews I conducted with survivors of those attacks, and the rescue workers involved in the response, and how important they were to me, not just for research, but also in terms of showcasing the lived reality of mental health.

I went into the disaster and mental health field without any prior knowledge, and without any clear guidance or advice inside my university (as disaster research and trauma research is, and this was the view of a committee in the aftermath of the attacks, poorly developed in Belgium). My own background is not at all in psychology, medicine, or anything similar. I studied sociology, followed by political sciences. Through a simple twist of fate, I came into this field, and knew I knew nothing about it, except that I loved it.

The interviews with the survivors, the rescue workers, those with—and those without—mental health issues are what formed my basis in mental health research. They were a scientific compass, which served me well even during my studies on COVID-19.

Later on, I found many more researchers with a similar mindset, trying to find a middle-way in trauma research, between the tunnel-vision psychological view and the blind literary view on trauma. Either way, that middle-way for me was found through those interviews; as such, my first acknowledgement needs to be to those survivors, family members, and rescue workers involved in the attacks of 22/03/2016 in Belgium.

Despite the academic lens of the book, I hope this book first and foremost represents a view of trauma that does not devolve into a form of *scientism*, and represents an attempt at showcasing the consequences of terrorism on us as human beings; sometimes from a birds-eye view, but also, I hope, from a grounded perspective.

Related to that "human perspective": this book was not written at all with Artificial Intelligence; not just out of principle, but also since my views collide at times with the majority opinion which AI always follows with regard to social sciences, and because I detest its vague writing style. My usage of ChatGPT limited itself to finding very specific articles that I could not find again, and that I was unable to find through scientific databases. Speaking of which, the magnificent PubMed was incredibly helpful in writing this book.

There are many, many other people I should thank. The relief of finishing the book would tempt one to thank everyone, but therefore perhaps thanking no one in particular. Hence, while of course I thank my friends and family, I have reserved this acknowledgement for a few people in particular.

Of course, I thank Springer Nature for the chance to write about the topic that captivated me for so many years, and allowing me an approach that focused less on psychological elements, and instead employed a quite pragmatic public health angle; and I thank of course specifically Janet Kim and Dhivya Savariraj for the editorial and production support.

My development as a researcher was very much dependent on several people. First, Johan Bilsen, thanks to whom I was able to finish my PhD after my first promotor had stopped caring about scientific research, who made sure I was always able to find some way to continue the research, and who supported my progress through my development as a researcher through more ways than I can name here.

Secondly, Lise Stene, with whom I wrote several articles, and with whom I worked during my stay at the Norwegian Centre for Violence and Traumatic Stress Studies in Norway. Most of my initial knowledge on public health interventions and psychosocial aid responses comes from Lise, and so Chap. 9 of this book no doubt carries a lot of Lise's scientific insights, or at least how I have learned about her insights.

I of course also thank my friends and family. Writing a book while working full time can be quite a time-consuming affair, and it helps to know there are people who care about what I do.

I specifically wish to thank my father for his never-ending support in my life, and my many academic and intellectual endeavours, as well as proofreading the chapter in which the Bhopal disaster is discussed and pointing out the technical error in my description of the disaster, as the chemical that was released was not a pesticide, but a product to make a pesticide. Additionally, I wrote this book mainly at his house, because my bathroom was being renovated, and I could not stay in my apartment in Ghent. I cannot thank him enough for both emotional and practical support.

Finally, I thank Nina, to whom this book is dedicated, and who, aside from her love and support, also gave me the motivation and courage to write this book. This book would not exist without her, and I cannot describe the happiness I feel in being able to dedicate this book to her. Even though this book is about the mental horrors humans can go through, she has made the process wonderful and unforgettable.

**Competing Interests** The author has no competing interests to declare that are relevant to the content of this manuscript.

# Contents

# About the Author

**Roel Van Overmeire, PhD** is a post-doctoral researcher at the Mental Health and Wellbeing Research Group (MENT) at the Vrije Universiteit Brussel in Belgium. His work has focused on mental health and terrorism, and he has published extensively on the mental health of survivors, the structural issues of the psychosocial response after terrorism, and theoretical discussions of post-traumatic stress disorder.

Beyond his research on terrorism, Roel Van Overmeire has explored diverse topics, such as mental health in patients with Parkinson's disease, psoriasis, and fibromyalgia; post-traumatic stress prevention after sexual assault; post-traumatic stress research during the pandemic; and the mental health effects of COVID-19 on funeral directors. He is a member of the Belgian Public Health Organization and the European Centre of Expertise for Victims of Terrorism, and has been a visiting researcher at the Norwegian Centre for Violence and Traumatic Stress Studies. His work has been presented at numerous conferences and has received coverage across Belgian media outlets.

# List of Abbreviations

| | |
|---|---|
| DSM | Diagnostic and Statistical Manual of Mental Disorders |
| FBI | Federal Bureau of Investigations |
| ICD | International Classification of Diseases |
| MDD | Major Depressive Disorder |
| MIC | Methyl-isocyanate |
| PHQ | Patient Health Questionnaire |
| PTG | Post-traumatic growth |
| PTSD | Post-traumatic stress disorder |
| UK | United Kingdom |
| U.N. | United Nations |
| U.S. | United States |

# Chapter 1
# Key Concepts in the Study of Mental Health After Terrorist Attacks

## 1.1 Researching Terrorism and Mental Health from a Public Health Perspective

The relationship between terrorism and mental health is a complex one. The difficulties arise from the get-go, namely at the conceptual level. What is terrorism? What is mental health? Both questions cannot be answered fully, because terrorism is in the eye of the beholder, and mental health is a very broad concept.

Therefore, what is important is that these concepts are discussed, and that it is explained what is meant by these concepts. It is namely impossible to discuss terrorism if it is not acknowledged that terrorism is very fluid concept, nor if the issues with measuring mental health are not discussed.

In addition, this is all done through the lens of public health. Thus, in the following sections, public health will be discussed, after which terrorism will be defined, and the link between public health and terrorism will be clarified. After this link is established, the research on terrorism and mental health will be discussed, as well as mental health concepts. The chapter ends with a methodological overview of terrorism research, providing information on the designs, scales, and other aspects of research.

---

Some of the content in this chapter is based on my doctoral thesis, defended in 2021. Van Overmeire, R. (2021). The association between exposure to terrorist attacks and mental health in Belgium. [PhD Thesis, Vrije Universiteit Brussel]. VUB Press. https://cris.vub.be/ws/portalfiles/portal/86873200/1_PDFsam_Van_Overmeire_Roel_PhD_thesis_20.12.2021.pdf



R. Van Overmeire, *Terrorism, Mental Health and Aftercare*,
https://doi.org/10.1007/978-3-032-31560-1_1

## 1.2 Public Health Perspective

Most studies on terrorism and mental health employ a public health perspective. Unfortunately, defining public health is equally difficult as terrorism and mental disorders [1].

To come to a definition, or description, there are some aspects that are roughly similar across differing definitions that can be combined. As such, public health *is a scientifically informed approach to improve and protect the health a community or population* [2–4]. This improvement and protection of the health can be achieved through preventive medicine, education, control of diseases, policy change, etc [2]. Considering the many ways in which this can be done, public health also consists of many different disciplines, such as epidemiology, biostatistics, biology, environmental sciences, behavioural and social sciences, and others [4].

The goal of public health is therefore a lot more practical than roughly sociology or psychology individually, where grand theory thinking informs practice more than in public health, where experience and observations generally do not create grand theories. Observation and experience are key to public health. Additionally, it is a jack of all trades that borrow techniques of specific disciplines, with as end goal the study and improvement of health, or in the case of this book, mental health.

**The Mandatory Illustration**

The classic example in every public health book to showcase the public health perspective is the example of a cholera outbreak in London in 1854. John Snow did not know the specificities of what cholera was but was able to locate the origin of the outbreak to a water pump. Once he discovered the source, the pump was closed and the cholera outbreak seceded [2]. It shows that exact knowledge of what a disease, or mental illness, constitutes off is not needed to take action in a public health approach. What is needed are observations and quick thinking; a sort of common-sense approach, coupled with pragmatism.

**Public Health or Public Mental Health?**

There has been a call from researchers to differentiate between public health and public *mental* health. Indeed, mental health has often been ignored in public health research, which is gap that needs to be filled [5, 6]. As one slogan of this movement goes: *there is no health without mental health* [7]. This book does not have "Public mental health" in its title as it seems inopportune to mend a lack of mental health by creating a separate section; if mental health is underrepresented, and essential to public health, then it seems better to see public health as always encompassing mental health.

## 1.3 Disasters

One typical area of intervention for public health is after disasters. Disasters are mass-scale events that can affect social structures and impact the usual functioning of a community or the society in which they take place. They often have physical consequences, but also psychological and psychosocial consequences [8–10].

Research on disasters with relation to mental health is difficult, due to the unexpected nature of disasters. It is difficult to predict when a disaster will strike; hence, preparing research to study the impact of a disaster on a population is an often chaotic, unprepared endeavour. This means that most studies will not have a clear pre-disaster measurement of a population (so, the mental health before the disaster strikes) and often a delay in the post-disaster measurement (e.g. due to needing to prepare how to gather the data among people affected).

**The First Disaster Studies**

Some of the first studies on mental health issues after disasters were conducted by a Swiss researcher named Edouard Stierlin. He was the first to compare man-made disasters with natural disasters and was a pioneer in investigating mental health issues are related to disaster exposure. For example, one of his studies showed that after the Messina earthquake in 1907 showed traumatic sleep disturbances for a considerable time among 25% of those exposed [11].

**Categorizing Disasters**

Disasters are generally divided into three large basic groups [12]:

1. Man-made disasters
2. Technological disasters
3. Natural disasters

Technological disasters are disasters such as the nuclear disaster at Chernobyl, while a natural disaster can be an earthquake or a famine [9, 10, 13]. However, natural disasters are often not purely natural disasters. Many are actually caused by human factors, such as famines or floods, who also often affect poor people more than other socio-economic classes [14]. The number of natural and technological disasters has increased over the years. For example, in 1992 there were 368 such disasters, while this was at average 650 for the period between 2004 and 2013 [15]. Man-made disasters are assumed to be the most distressing [10, 12], and can be mass-shooting, or the subject of this book: terrorist attacks [16].

## 1.4 Terrorism

The paradox of terrorism is that everyone knows what terrorism is, and at the same time, everyone disagrees on what terrorism is, or in other words, political sciences nor nations have come to a consensus of what terrorism is [17].

On a nation level, there is the issue that terrorism is the eye of the beholder; while it is a cliché that terrorism-researcher have heard one too many times, it is true that one nation's terrorist is another's freedom fighter [18]. For example, the Irish Republican Army's bombing would be seen as act of resistance by some in Northern Ireland, and terrorism by the British government. From the Soviet Union's perspective, the Muhaiyaddeen were terrorists, from American perspective freedom fighters.

It might seem therefore that nations simply want to be able to call anyone and not be restricted by semantics. However, it has a specific legal dimension as well, as what one can legally call internationally terrorism is of course important: a plane hijacking can be due to ordinary crime (e.g. wanting a ransom—as was the case in the majority of cases before 9/11) or terrorist in nature (e.g. the 9/11 attacks). The United Nations (UN) discussions on defining terrorism are interesting in this respect. For example, there was a consensus in the UN on the bare minimum, namely that certain armed activities can be considered terrorist:

> Acts intended or calculated to provoke a state of terror in the general public, a group of persons or particular persons for political purposes are in any circumstance unjustifiable, whatever the considerations of a political, philosophical, ideological, racial, ethnic, religious or any other nature that may be invoked to justify them [19].

Yet, while this is a consensus, it doesn't show a definition as such. In fact, most anti-terrorism instruments do not contain any form of definition of terrorism, due to the political sensitivity [19].

Even ignoring the political agendas, it is difficult to find a definition in political sciences, or better put, finding one definition is easy; finding one everyone agrees with is nigh impossible.

There are two main philosophically different ways of looking at the issue: some have adhered to the subjectivist view, namely that terrorism is in the eye of the beholder, as mentioned earlier, and thus a definition should depend on the need of a nation [20, 21]. Others have tried to find an objective basis of what terrorism constitutes off, with the reasoning that fighting terrorism is impossible if there is no shared idea of it [20]. The issues are however many in this approach as well. For example, how can terrorism be differentiated from other forms of violence. Schmid [22] summarizes how defining terrorism can be approached. It can be done through a historical lens, a psychological lens, a differentiation with other forms of violence (e.g. violent crime), or focusing on the terrorist attack in itself.

However, each focus has its issues.

When summarizing in what all definition overlap, it seems that over 80% agree that terrorism has an aspect of violence, but that is the most agreement that can be found. It is seen as political in 65% of the definitions, but the element of fear and terror, that some see as essential, is only found in 51% of the definitions [18, 22].

For example, while some see terrorism as the acts aimed at destabilizing a society through fear caused by violence, by organizations that are spread around the world and have a broad ideological goal [23], the Federal Bureau of Investigations simply removes that "fear" factor: "*Violent, criminal acts committed by individuals and/or groups to further ideological goals stemming from domestic influences, such as those of a political, religious, social, racial, or environmental nature.*" [24].

A major problem in the field is that (1) it makes large generalizations out of anecdotal evidence [18]; (2) it causes empirical limitations to itself. The first point is obvious: terrorism is not so common. As will be argued towards the end of this chapter, it is precisely because it is so uncommon in the West, that it mainly studied in the West.

Secondly, a clear example of empirical limitations is the earlier mentioned "fear" factor. Half of the definitions have the idea that the goal of terrorism is to cause fear or cause change through fear [18], yet it is simply impossible to prove this. For example, the attacks in Belgium were executed by suicide bombers: how can one check if these people aimed at causing fear or wanted change in society through fear? In fact, the definition also holds back calling something terrorism until the aspect of fear has been proven.

It reminds one of the philosophies of George Berkelley, who stated that "esse est percipi": to be is to be perceived [25]; or in other words (to quote on the thought experiments misattributed to him): if a tree falls in the forest and no one is around to hear it, does it make a sound? Or: if a terrorist attack takes place, and there is no one around to tell you it was intended to cause fear, is it a terrorist attack? If not, according to the "fear" definition of terrorism, the terrorist attack never happens; just like the tree never made a sound. The "fear" element is inherently unobservable, just like the tree falling without no one around is inherently unobservable.

Berkeley solved the problem of the tree with God: God sees all, therefore, the tree is observed to fall and therefore makes a sound. In the case of terrorist attacks, it seems this role is fulfilled by political scientists: it is a terrorist attack, because they assign it to be as such. Clearly, that is not the ideal solution, but it is unfortunately necessary to move forward with this lacking concept, because the goal in this book is not that discussion, but the consequences of terrorism.

**Waves of Terrorism**

Terrorism is nothing new [18]. The Jewish Sicarri sect, which used suicide attacks against the Romans, and in Medieval times, the notorious Assassin sect which used public knife attacks to terrorize communities, are just two examples of the long history of terrorism [26, 27].

Modern terrorism is situated to begin in the late nineteenth century, and is divided into four waves following the framework of Rapoport [23].

1. The Anarchist wave, starting in the late nineteenth century, was, as the name indicates, led by Anarchist terrorist, and arguably best exemplified with the assassination of Tsar Nicolas I of Russia in 1881, the assassination of United States president William McKinley in 1901, and the Wall Street bombing in 1920.

2. The anticolonial wave, beginning in the 1920s, and ending around 40 years later. It followed the treaty of Versailles, and the call of the United States, and Woodrow Wilson for "self-determination" [28].
3. The New Left Wave, which can be characterized by terrorist organisations such as the Rote *Armee Fraktion* in Germany, the *Brigate Rose* in Italy or The Weatherman in the United States. Arguably the most infamous incident was the kidnapping of Italian Prime Minister Aldo Moro, who eventually was killed when the government refused to negotiate.
4. The Religious wave, which is characterized by not just Islamic extremist attacks, but also the Japanese Sarin attacks, or the Oklahoma City Bombing [18]. The Religious wave started around the 1970s and has Islam at the heart of it [23]. To provide some more context, a short section of Islamic terrorism.

**Islamic Terrorism**

Modern day extremist Islamic terrorism can be, as always "arguably," traced back to the Islamic Sunni thinker Sayyid Qutb, who (disillusioned and disgusted by what he saw as the materialism and decadence of the United States, as well disappointed with what he saw as the return to paganism of the Islamic world) called for violent jihad [29]. Al-Qaeda leaders saw him as an inspiration, and Osama bin Laden attended the lessons of Qutb's brother Muhammed [29, 30].

The basis of suicide bombing was created by Shiite terrorists during the Lebanese civil war. In 1983, a terrorist exploded his yellow Mercedes truck, killing American soldiers in Beirut, who were stationed there as peacekeeping force. The death toll of 241 killed soldiers was the largest loss since Iwo Jima in 1945 [30]. Since then, the tactics of the Shiite terrorists have been copied by many different terrorist groups, including al-Qaeda, eventually resulting in the attacks of 11 September 2001 [29, 30], yet the field of terrorism and mental health research did not kickstart after these attacks—in fact, it was anti-government attack, which was also part of the religious wave of terrorist attacks.

## 1.5 Terrorism and Mental Health Research

In 1995, two American citizens sought revenge against the United States government, after an FBI intervention in the town Waco had gone wrong. The FBI had laid siege on a compound of a local cult, called the Branch Davidians, in Waco. The siege ended with 76 people dying in a firefight and the explosion of the compound. McVie and Nichols, in an act of revenge, bombed a federal building in Oklahoma City, killing 168 people. It was the largest attack on United States territory since Pearl Harbour in 1941. While it was only after 9/11 that the study of terrorism and mental health began to boom [31], the foundation had been made by the studies in Oklahoma-City. Naturally, there had been studies before these, but these were relatively few and sparse (see e.g. [32]).

In this section, certain technical aspects of these studies will be discussed in short, as these are relevant for the further discussion throughout the book.

### *1.5.1 Exposure*

There are two ways to view the link between terrorism and mental health. First, through direct exposure. *Direct exposure* is often defined quite loosely, though one can view it as is done in criterion A of post-traumatic stress disorder (PTSD) in the Diagnostic and Statistical Manual of Mental Disorders (DSM)-5 [33]. Thus, direct exposure to terrorist attacks is:

1. Experiencing an attack first hand, meaning being present at the event when it happens.
2. Losing a close family member, significant other, or close friend in the terrorist attack without being present.
3. Working in the aftermath of the terrorist attack, in that the person sees the remains of people—this will apply mostly to rescue workers (e.g. fireman or nurses) [34].

The second way to view the link is as *indirect exposure*. This is essentially every form of exposure that is not covered by direct exposure, which can constitute as viewing a terrorist attack through media, or hearing about the attacks from someone else, etc., yet this does not exclude that this person might experience stress or mental health issues. In this case, researchers will look at the impact of terrorism in a different way. Suicides, heart attacks, perception of threat, and media-viewing are all different indicators aside from direct exposure [34].

## 1.6 Mental Health

This exposure to terrorism can be associated with certain mental health outcomes. The World Health Organization defines mental health as "*Mental health is a state of mental well-being that enables people to cope with the stresses of life, realize their abilities, learn well and work well, and contribute to their community. It has intrinsic and instrumental value and is integral to our well-being*" [35].

There are of course many other definitions in this case as well, such as "*the successful performance of mental function, resulting in productive activities, fulfilling relationships, the ability to adapt to change and successful coping with adversity*" [36].

Either way, when there are issues with mental health, this can be in the form of what is called mental disorders. Examples of mental disorders are post-traumatic stress disorder, major depression, anxiety disorder… Besides an effect on the mental state, the behavioural state can also be affected of someone who such a disorder

[33, 34, 37]. Note that these disorders are a form of systematic grouping of symptoms. For example, feeling bad or down is not a mental disorder, but it can be a symptom of one. Developing mental disorders significantly lowers the years lived without disability and even the average years lived overall [38]. For example, one of the largest burdens of disease worldwide is depression, and people with depression have a much higher risk of dying from natural causes or suicide, and have an all-round higher mortality [34, 39, 40].

The consequences of having a disorder can be wide-reaching, such as job loss, poverty, suicide, etc [41]. Depression, for example, has a huge economic impact. Beside the impact of the person with depression, studies show that depression can have an impact on the economy at large: the treatment of MDD is estimated to have cost the US$210 billion, and in England, only for the direct treatment of MDD, 370 million pounds [42].

Mental disorders can also be related to stigmatization, and people with mental disorders might be excluded from public life, political life, and/or abused, both verbally as well as physically and sexually [43, 44]. In low or middle-income countries, the overwhelming majority of people with disorders are not treated, yet, even in high-income countries half of the people with disorders can remain untreated [45, 46]. This is also the case for victims of terrorism, who often do not get the necessary help, and this even 10–15 years after the event [34, 47–50].

**Mental Illness and Insanity**

In the nineteenth century, a major difference was made between insanity and mental illness, often characterized in the form of hysteria (nicknamed "the female malady", as it was associated with being female, and when diagnosed in men seen as being especially shameful for them).

This difference between insanity and hysteria was often class-based, and gender based. For example, in his book on hysteria, the surgeon Sir Benjamin Brodie states "*I do not hesitate to declare that among the higher classes of society, at least four fifths of the female patients, who are commonly supposed to labour under diseases of the joints, labour under hysteria, and nothing else*" [51].

Another example of the importance of this difference is found in the writings of one Dr. Mayo, who describes in his collection of lectures called "Medical Testimony and Evidence in Cases of Lunacy" the case of, the very clearly rich, Ms. Cummins. Dr. Mayo states that Ms. Cummins was surely ill, but not insane, as she did not hear voices, nor saw anything that was not there. However, she did give 2000 pounds to someone not equipped for it, and she had been screaming, causing the police to come to her, despite there being no danger [52].

It was better to be hysterical, or have any of the other high-class diseases (such as neurasthenia), than to be insane, because that meant going to institutions.

– Diagnostical Manuals

There are two main diagnostical systems in which mental disorders are described: Diagnostic and Statistical Manual of Mental Disorders (DSM) and the International Classification of Diseases (ICD).[1]

The DSM has two periods of existence. Originally, it was Freudian inspired, until 1980, when the American Psychiatric Association broke with the Freudian influence (almost) completely, and focused on a Kraepelinian biomedical system (there is a certain irony here, since Freud was, reportedly, envious of Kraepelin) [53, 54]. The main difference between both systems comes down to the "meaning" of symptoms. In a Freudian system, symptoms have causes; in a Kraepelinian system, in imitation of diagnostic systems for physical health, symptoms stand on their own, and do not need a cause. That meant that a mental disorder could be described as one would cancer or the flu.

In the following sections, the triumvirate of mental disorders will be discussed, namely depressive disorder, anxiety disorder and PTSD. These are a triumvirate for two reasons:

1. Because they are simply the most studied in terrorism and mental health studies, which is not surprising, since PTSD is linked with disaster-research due to its nature, and depression and anxiety are so common.
2. Because the overlap between these three disorders is large, and correlations between them are often quite large.

For all these disorders, it is important to note that they all have the classification that they can only be diagnosed if they actually cause functional or social impairment. For example, criterion B in major depressive disorder, criterion H in PTSD, and criterion D in generalized anxiety disorder all read:

> The symptoms cause clinically significant distress or impairment in social, occupational, or other important areas of functioning [33].

Furthermore, each disorder also has other criteria outside the symptom criteria, such as that the symptoms cannot be related to drug abuse or other mental disorders [33].

## *1.6.1 Depression*

Historically, depression as mental health issue is old, with references to it in one way or another dating back to ancient times; though, it must be added that the symptoms changed radically throughout time (e.g. much more physically focused), and it is only in the twentieth century that the diagnosis became quite stable [55].

[1] The ICD also describes general diseases, such as cancer and other diseases.

Major depressive disorder (MDD) is one of the most common disorders in the world [56–58]. Despite there being differences in symptoms depending on the country and culture [59], it is relative stable diagnosis, as it has remained relatively unchanged in each iteration of the ICD and DSM [60, 61]. The disorder has several aspects. First, it consists of five or more symptoms during a 2-week period. The most well-known symptom is having a depressed mood most of the day. To be diagnosed with MDD, at least one of two symptoms need to be present: depressed mood or loss of interest/pleasure [33]. Other symptoms can include weight loss, insomnia, hypersomnia, fatigue or loss of energy, feelings of worthlessness, diminished ability to think or concentrate or reoccurring thoughts of death (e.g. suicidal ideation) [34, 60]. There are 227 possible ways in which someone might have MDD, showcasing the large heterogeneity of the disorder, and meaning in practice that 227 people with MDD, could all have slightly different forms of MDD [62].

### *1.6.2 Anxiety*

Fear and anxiety are important parts of how we survive as a species. While fear and anxiety overlap, the difference is that fear occurs when there is a real or perceived imminent threat, while anxiety is the anticipation of future threat [33]. When this anxiety is regular, arises without identifiable trigger, and comprises daily life, there is reason to suspect it concerns an anxiety disorder [63, 64].

While there are different types of anxiety disorders, there is a type of anxiety disorder that applies to general anxiety, namely generalized anxiety disorder. A generalized anxiety disorder is characterized by excessive worrying and worry for more than 6 months that is difficult to control, and three of the following symptoms: restlessness or feeling keyed up or on edge, being easily fatigued, difficulty concentrating or one's mind going blank, irritability, muscle tension, and sleep disturbance. As with all disorders, the symptoms must impair the daily functioning of the person, and should not be caused by substances, and not be better explained by another disorder [33, 34].

With a prevalence rate between 20% and 33%, anxiety disorders can be considered common worldwide [63, 64], though when looking at specific anxiety disorders, such as generalized anxiety disorder, the prevalence is around 2–6% [33, 64, 65]. This worldwide prevalence is also uneven worldwide, with women and people in developed countries developing it more than people from the Global South [33, 34].

### *1.6.3 Post-traumatic Stress Disorder*

PTSD is a trauma- and stressor-related disorder, described in both the DSM-5 and the ICD-11 [33, 37]. As the majority of studies in terrorism follow the DSM definition, this one will be expanded on—since the definition do differ quite a bit between the DSM and the ICD, as will be discussed later.

However, even within the DSM there are some differences between the DSM-IV and the DSM-5 definition. Even the categorization of PTSD was different in the DSM-IV, where it was seen as an anxiety disorder, while in the DSM-5 it is a trauma and stressor-related disorder [33, 66]. That PTSD was seen as an anxiety-related disorder makes sense, considering its overlap in symptoms with anxiety, but also depression [67]. For clarity, the major differences between DSM-IV and DSM-5 will be ignored in describing the symptoms of PTSD.

PTSD is a mental disorder that can arise as a consequence of exposure to trauma (this is the co-called criterion A), and can lead to symptoms that are divided into different criteria (which need to be met to get a diagnosis):

- Criterion B: intrusion, such as involuntary distress memories or dreams, or flashbacks
- Criterion C: avoidance, such as avoidance of distressing memories
- Criterion D: negative alterations, such as detachment, having very negative beliefs about oneself or the world
- Criterion E: alterations in arousal and reactivity, meaning for example reckless behaviour, or concentration issues, or hypervigilance

These symptoms must last 1 month.

What is worthwhile to note is that there is such a variation in possibilities of symptom combination, that there are in total 636,120 different possible symptom combinations that make "post-traumatic stress disorder" [68]. In other words, there is anything but a uniform PTSD experience.

Overall, PTSD appears roughly the same all over the world. There are exceptions, for example the inability inability to recall specific aspects of the trauma and blame of self or others for the event, that are not so globally common, and in some cultures, symptoms appear with PTSD that do not appear in the diagnostical criteria of PTSD [69].

**Short History of Trauma**

While PTSD occurs more or less across the world, there is surprisingly little evidence of it occurring throughout time. Several writers have tried to find evidence of it in ancient times, or is even mentioned in the Bible, the Iliad, or even Shakespeare [70, 71]. For example, in Henry IV, some assume that when Lady Percy describes the deteriorating king's emotional condition, describing his nightmares, she is describing PTSD [68], yet actual evidence is slim, as oftentimes passages do not really describe PTSD, but stress reactions during battle, or fear and sadness shortly after battle. Furthermore, there is such a desire to find PTSD throughout history, that someone with nightmares of war is immediately seen as having PTSD. This seems quite unjustified.

That does not mean also that there were no mental health issues related to war. For example, by the end of the Roman republic, until the late Roman empire, there was certainly attention for the mental health of Roman soldiers, and it seems that soldiers with mental health problems were a regular sight [72]. However, definitive evidence of PTSD in ancient times simply does not exist [73].

(continued)

**(continued)**

Starting in the nineteenth century, there are the first clear descriptions of things one would recognize as somewhat reminiscent of the present-day PTSD. For example Herbert Page wrote down his observations of some patients after train accidents: "*It is this same element of fear which in railway collisions has so large a share […] The incidents indeed of almost every railway collision are quite sufficient—even if no bodily injury be inflicted—to produce a very serious effect upon the mind, and to be the means of bringing about a state of collapse from fright, and from fright only*" [74].

These mental reactions to severe stress have been known under many different names starting in the nineteenth century: "le vent du boulet" ("wind of the cannonball"—a condition among soldiers during the Napoleonic wars), "soldier's heart" (among soldiers during the American Civil War) [73], "the engineer's malady" (due to the high amount of stress on train drivers due to the high amount of train accidents in the nineteenth century) [75], railway spine (named after train passengers who experienced anxiety after train accidents) [11], shellshock (during the First World War) [75], etc.

The origin of the term "trauma," or "psychological trauma," also comes from the nineteenth century. Mental health was mainly viewed in physiological terms [11, 54, 76]. For example, the severe anxiety people showed after a train accident was seen by some as being a severe emotional blow to the spine.

It is based on such ideas that Hermann Oppenheim stated that survivors of industrial incidents with mental health issues (or what one would now classify as mental health issues) had physical injuries, though with a certain psychological issue underneath as well. He called it "traumatic neuroses"—the first mention of psychological trauma was a type of trauma that combined both physical and psychological causes [68].

The famous neurologist Jean-Martin Charcot tried his hand in explaining the hysteria from this perspective as well, but failed. Another neurologist, Sigmund Freud (an admirer of Charcot) followed with his attempt at curing, or at least understanding, hysteria. Sigmund Freud, in his early writings together with Josef Breuer, provided a basis of what trauma is understood to be now, based on earlier work of Pierre Janet [11]. In his studies on patients with hysteria, they hypothesized that patients were overwhelmed with fright, leading to a sort of traumatic helplessness; as such, fear caused a traumatic neurosis [11]. Indeed, that meant that anyone could suffer from such traumatic neurosis, which was an important break with the nineteenth century thinking of hereditary neurosis, but also a break with the physiological thinking towards a psychological thinking [54].

(continued)

**(continued)**

In the case of hysteria, this would have been sexual experiences in childhood. As Freud wrote "*I therefore put forward the thesis that at the bottom of every case of hysteria there are one or more occurrences of premature sexual experience*" [77].

However, the problem, as described by Judith Herman, was that so many women had hysteria—meaning that many of the high-class women of society would have had sexual trauma in their childhood [16]. Not only that, but he was also never able to prove that any patients actually had experienced sexual trauma in childhood [54]. Thus, he buried his so-called seduction theory, and, in Herman's words, "*Out of the ruins of the traumatic theory of hysteria, Freud created psychoanalysis*" [16]. As such, Freud's work started to concentrate more on the internal than any external factor [11, 16, 54].

Indeed, as Carl Jung had written of Freud: he broke with the nineteenth century, but did not know what to break through to something new [78]. What did bring in twentieth century thought about trauma, was the other break with the nineteenth century: the First World War [79].

It is through the war that trauma becomes *psychological* trauma (e.g. shellshock); though, as has been noted, every instance of description of trauma and its reactions has had precedents in the nineteenth century [80]. For example, the many shellshocked soldiers of the First World War forced Freud to, yet again, revise his idea of trauma, making it into an external event that is unexpected and overwhelming in its nature [54], thereby somewhat repeating earlier observations of nineteenth century doctors such Herbert Page on survivors of railway accidents [74]. While this pivot in Freud's thinking did not really affect his general psychoanalytical theory, it did form the basis of the future DSM-III definition of trauma [54].

**Difference with the ICD-11 PTSD Definition**

The ICD-11 has a slightly different approach to PTSD. It also requires an exposure to an event, described as "extremely threatening or horrific event or series of events," while in the DSM-5, criterion A of PTSD, this is described more extensively: "*Exposure to actual or threatened death, serious injury, or sexual violence,*" after which several possibilities are stated, such as directly witnessing the event, or experiencing the horrific details of the aftermath of a trauma (e.g. medical personnel who have to treat victims of a terrorist attack) [33, 37].

What is very different from the DSM-5 definition is that the ICD-11 also includes a "PTSD-plus": complex PTSD. This can only occur after "*exposure to an event or series of events of an extremely threatening or horrific nature, most commonly prolonged or repetitive events from which escape is difficult or impossible (e.g. torture, slavery, genocide campaigns, prolonged domestic violence, repeated childhood sexual or physical abuse).*" [37] The DSM-5, nor any DSM, has this differentiation, and it is assumed that the DSM definition also contains such trauma exposure.

However, there is an issue with the trauma indicator in the DSM either way, which has nothing to do with the ICD-11.

**The Issue with the Traumatic Event Indicator**

PTSD is an oddity compared to most disorders, in the sense that it is not purely a symptom-based disorder, but a disorder that can only be diagnosed when certain social conditions have been met. Concretely, in the DMS-5, PTSD is divided into different criteria that have been explained earlier, most of which are symptom criteria. However, the first criterion is, as mentioned, criterion A, which indicates the "trauma exposure."

This point is also true for ICD-11 [81]. The ICD-11 sees traumatic events as the exposure to "*an extremely threatening or horrific event or series of events*" [37].

As can be noted, the trauma exposure definition does not include, nor imply, symptoms. In fact, diagnostically speaking, to have post-traumatic symptoms, a person must first have experienced something that fits the definition of trauma [34, 37]. It is important to stress that this trauma does not, in itself, indicate that someone will have symptoms; in other words, one can fulfill criterion A without actually having any symptoms at all. This is in stark difference with the DSM-IV, where having experienced a trauma only fulfilled criterion A if it was *also* coupled with feelings of shame, fear, and helplessness.

However, that caused methodological issues: if a trauma is only a trauma if it causes shame, fear and helplessness, at what point do these emotional reactions become *post*-traumatic stress [82]? Or in other words, one could argue that the DSM-IV explained *symptoms on the basis of symptoms*, as shame, fear, and helplessness are also symptoms of PTSD, while also being a requisite for fulfilling criterion A [83]. This simply to showcase the importance of differentiating the trauma (e.g. the event) and the symptoms from a theoretical and diagnostic point of view [81]. It is also why criterion A or the traumatic event indicator in the ICD-11 have been called "gate keepers": one needs to go through the metaphorical gate (e.g. fulfilling the trauma indicator) before the PTSD-like symptoms they have can be called "PTSD" [84, 85].

However, most studies using PTSD have not used any form of trauma-indicator. For example, during the COVID-19 pandemic, only roughly 10% of the studies on PTSD used any form of trauma indicator [84]. This was because many of these studies assumed that that anyone living during the corona pandemic was exposed to trauma, yet, because COVID-19 studies did not use a trauma indicator, many of these studies did not differentiate between common stress, adjustment disorder (a stress-related disorder), and PTSD, nor did it differentiate between those who are bored at their house, those who are being abused during their isolation, and those who are simply stressed due to their work [84, 85].

This is also true for terrorism studies. Most terrorism studies have always assumed that anyone who experienced terrorism fits the trauma-indicator, but also, that terrorism caused all the symptoms they experience [31]. However, some terrorism studies show that this is certainly not the case, whether it is among survivors of bombing in Northern Ireland, or survivors in Pakistan, the event to which they relate symptoms is not always the terrorist attack they experienced [86, 87]. In short, terrorism studies, generally, suffer from a form of tunnel vision, wherein only the terrorist attack can "explain" the symptoms [31].

**Partial/Subthreshold PTSD**

While PTSD in the DSM does not have a differentiation in terms of PTSD and complex PTSD, researchers using the DSM definition have made their own differentiations. The most common of these is partial PTSD, or subthreshold PTSD (these terms are used for the same idea; one study after the Paris attacks for example studies partial PTSD, but to explain it references a study using subthreshold PTSD [88]). Partial/subthreshold PTSD is PTSD that does not fulfil the requirements for "full-on" PTSD completely [89]. It has been argued that such partial/subthreshold PTSD holds value in showcasing people who do not completely fulfil PTSD criteria, but still suffer from severe mental health issues [89].

In this book, partial PTSD will be ignored, for the simple reason that PTSD in itself is already being overestimated due to research design choices, which is the topic of the next section, and thus would not add extra information to the reader—and in fact, adding partial PTSD to the discussion would cause more issues, since there are multiple definitions of what partial/subthreshold PTSD should look like.

## 1.7 Measuring Mental Health Issues After Terrorism

Studies on mental health after terrorism can come in many forms. However, most do follow a similar pattern [31].

### *1.7.1 Research Design*

Research designs are the approach a researcher takes to answer their research question. Terrorism studies do this in two forms: qualitative and quantitative.

**Quantitative**

Quantitative designs are focussed on collecting data on as many people as relevant, and, generally, having this data in the form of numeric outcomes [90]. The most common form, in terrorism research, is do this in a so-called cross-sectional design. A cross-sectional design is a one-time measurement, meaning that there is no further follow-up of someone who provided data. For example, participants in a study on an early study after 9/11 were called up, but after this never contacted again for a study looking at how their mental health state was later on in their lives [91]. Naturally, such studies are limited in what they can say. For example, what is often important in terrorism studies is to know whether or not mental health symptoms dissipate or increase.

However, with only one measurement, it is unclear in what way the measurement is a good reflection of how many of those people will have mental health issues later on.

There are studies that look at the long-term impact. However, this is not always "longitudinal" in the sense that participants of the first measurements are not always included in the second measurement. This is often quite difficult to achieve, since it requires close follow-up of participants of the first measurement as to include them in the studies.

**Qualitative**

Qualitative research is another approach compared to quantitative designs, wherein the aim is not the amount of data that is collected, but the depth of the data [90, 92]. This can come in the form of interviews or focus groups (e.g. multiple participants together at the same time). The reason for doing such research can be because there are some aspects that quantitative research has difficulties figuring out. For example, a study in Belgium after the 2016 attack showcased the issues employees experienced in the post-attack workplace. While this could have been approached with pre-made questions, where an employee can answer from 1 to 5 how happy they are in their place, it would not have given information on the reason behind the answer. Thus, this qualitative study had a more in-depth look of the issues, many of which only became know because of the research, and thus could not have been included in a survey beforehand [93].

However, qualitative research is rare in terrorism studies—or disaster studies in general [94].

### *1.7.2 Measurements*

The majority of measurements in surveys in these terrorism studies are, not surprisingly, mental health scales. These often appear in the form of so-called Likert scales. Likert scales are, probably, the most used scales in disaster research. They appear in the form of a question (or statement), followed by a scale with five or ten options indicating agreement or disagreement [95]. A mental health measurement can focus on general health or focus on specific mental disorders.

**Screening**

Such scales are most commonly administrated through surveys, through a so-called self-report. Self-reported surveys are thought to lead to higher estimates than clinical interviews [96]. In general, the gold standard is therefore clinical interviews. A clinical interview however is expensive, considering it means that someone trained to take questionnaires is paid, and it takes a lot more time. It is therefore no surprise that the overwhelming majority of studies in terrorism are so-called self-report survey [31]. Self-report studies are studies where the sample that is being studied, answers questions about their mental health and other aspects by themselves—hence, the name "self-reported." For example, a classic survey is the "satisfaction survey" of large companies: when you have bought something, the company wants to know your opinion about the product you bought through the means of a survey.

Self-report surveys are quite common in disaster studies, and this is often due to practical reasons: it is easier to get a larger sample with self-reported questionnaires, cheaper, and less time intensive. The pragmatism of self-reported studies is also clear in the observation that most studies during the pandemic were also self-reported: while most countries had severe restrictions, self-reported online surveys were a way of collecting data [84].

A common critique on terrorism studies is this overreliance on self-reported studies [31]. It is impossible, from a psychological/psychiatric viewpoint, to diagnose any disorder through self-report; a professional needs to diagnose this. As such, a self-report study can only "screen" for mental health issues: they are estimates, not diagnoses [97]. As such, self-report studies do not match the outcomes of clinical interviews [98]. Hence also why screening studies cannot, nor are expected to, take into account all elements necessary to estimate a disorder in a population. For example, the Patient-Health Questionnaire-9, a typical depression-measurement, screens for all nine symptoms of the DSM-5 definition, yet it is often taken without the specification that at least one of two symptoms need to be present, namely depressed mood or loss of interest/pleasure [33]. Most screening studies simply take a sum score of the PHQ-9, meaning, someone might not have any depressed mood nor loss of interest/pleasure, and still score high on the PHQ-9 and be seen as having depression. Additionally, MDD actually has more criteria. Criterion B states "*The symptoms cause clinically significant distress or impairment in social, occupational, or other important areas of functioning.*" [33] This is seldom measured, since it is often assumed symptoms do that.

However, studies show that clinical interviews are not by definition better. For example, some interviewers in this gold standard are not trained as interviewers, or might not know enough about the specific mental health disorder they are meant to investigate [99]. Furthermore, studies show that self-report can be as good as clinical interviews [100–102], with one study on borderline personality disorder suggesting that a combination of both self-report and clinical interviews is better [103, 104]. However, there are major exceptions.

**Self-Report and Tunnel Vision**

The issue in disaster studies is not the focus on self-report; it is that the self-report is used to do half-measures. Specifically in measuring PTSD, self-report oriented studies often neglect to measure criterion A [31, 84, 105]. The solution many of these studies employ is to use "implied" exposure, meaning that when people answer a PTSD-scale, it is assumed they are referring to a terrorist attack—thus, there is no need to measure criterion A. For example, one study on terrorism in Israel states: "*We deemed it important to examine all participants as virtually everyone in Israel has at least vicarious exposure to terrorism*" [106]. This is a widespread problem in terrorism studies and other disaster fields (e.g. corona pandemic) [31, 84].

There are huge differences when criterion A is assessed and when it is not. For example, one study during the Second Intifada showed that the difference of assessing PTSD in the population with and without criterion A is 0.5% when measured in a clinical interview, and 9% when measured through self-report. In fact, self-report can be more than 40% higher than a clinical interview when not assessing trauma exposure [107–109]. This is not to point out that clinical interviews should be used—as mentioned, they are certainly not perfect, costly, and slow [107]. It is to point out that the combination of PTSD and self-report has led to PTSD estimations that are very far removed from diagnostical realities. This neglect of measuring criterion A had led to rampant increases in PTSD percentages that become nigh useless, reaching percentages of over 90% in for example one study [110]. From a public health perspective: what does public health policy do with studies that say that almost everyone has PTSD?

Though a repetition of what has been mentioned in an earlier section, it bears repeating: without the criterion A assessment, it is very unclear in relation to what respondents are answering. Most PTSD-scales ask the respondent to think about their most stressful event. They are given a list of so-called life-events, or are free to write the event themselves. After this, they are asked to respond to the symptom part of the PTSD-questionnaire, and relate the questions on symptoms to the event they indicated [84]. It can therefore be that their most stressful event was a divorce, an exam, sexual assault, breaking their leg, etc. The inability to assess the trauma defeats the purpose of assessing post-*traumatic* stress.

## 1.8 The Focus of Terrorism Studies

Most terrorism studies are concerned with survivors of terrorism. As Chap. 2 will show, there is a wealth of evidence of the association between mental health and being exposed to a terrorist attack. The majority of studies are performed through quantitative cross-sectional designs, though Belgian research on terrorism has employed qualitative designs more compared to the total output of their terrorism studies.

With regard to mental health, the focus is PTSD, where the majority of studies have studied PTSD, often in combination with anxiety or depression [31]. Almost all studies use the DSM-IV or DSM-5 definitions. In general, DSM-IV definitions were used a lot because it was the most recent DSM version at the time of studies—as the DSM-5 only came out in 2013. Furthermore, some studies have continued to use the DSM-IV for longitudinal reasons, as to ensure data is comparable.

Following this, there are also differences between countries that study mental health after terrorism. One notable aspect is the earlier mention partial/subthreshold PTSD: while French studies will generally use these, Norwegian studies often use this less.

Finally, most studies are concerned with mental health after extremist Islamic terrorism. For example, all 2010s French studies, Belgian studies, and almost all American studies, are on Islamic terrorist attacks. However, there is also a growing field focussing on religious/nationalist terrorist attacks, whether in Norway after the Utoya attacks, or studies on the Christchurch attacks.

## 1.9 Geographical Location of Most Terrorism Studies

While terrorism is a global phenomenon, the research on terrorism is a mostly Western affair [111]. This is even more so for mental health studies on terrorism. The majority of studies come from the United States and Israel, while France, Norway, the United Kingdom, New-Zealand, and other European countries provide most of the other studies. There are a few studies from Turkey or Pakistan (e.g. [86, 112–114]), but these are the exception to the rule, yet, most attacks do not occur in the United States, nor France, and Norway. Israel is, in fact, the only country where it seems that the many mental health studies make sense in association with the number of terrorist attacks it endures.

It seems that most countries do not have the cultural focus or fear for terrorism that leads to (1) the establishment of organisations that study terrorism; (2) to the study of the effects of terrorism on society or survivors. This is certainly not the case for other disasters. China published the second most PTSD-studies in the world during the corona pandemic [84], while Turkey has published extensively on the 2023 Kahramanmaraş earthquakes [115]. It furthermore is clear that it is not an issue of funding. There are well-executed studies in region torn apart by war, such as Myanmar [116], Afghanistan [117], Ethiopia [118], and others that will be further discussed in a later chapter. In fact, natural and technological disaster research and studies on war are performed globally—terrorism research simply is not.

The cultural fear of terrorist attacks seems to be larger in the West. This might also be partly because of 9/11; the restrictions it brought along were mainly Western, and led to two major wars in Afghanistan and Iraq that also brought troops in action ranging from the United States to Denmark to the United Kingdom. Terrorism has, perhaps paradoxically, a sort of exceptionalism to it: in societies that are overall relatively safe, it might feel as more important and more likely to happen than it actually does. In the terms of the sociologist Ulrich Beck, the modern West is a risk society, where everything is calculated in risks, and where very unlikely events are the ones that are seen to have the biggest impact, precisely because of their unlikeliness [119].

In public health terms, this is shown in the vulnerability paradox. Countries that are more vulnerable to disasters, whether natural or man-made, have much lower PTSD-rates than countries that are not vulnerable [120]. In other words, Western countries that are generally safe, are, on country level, more prone to developing

PTSD in the population when a disaster does strike. The same observation was found for suicide [121].

In addition, Western countries are much more under the influence of psychiatric thinking [122]. As authors have pointed out, sadness has been transformed into prolonged grief or depressive disorder [123]. Related to this, the democratic liberal countries also have more a cultural inclination towards "victimhood" [124]. For example, the idea of "microaggressions" is a "quick" way to victimhood. Victimhood is celebrated in, mostly, democratic countries; while other cultures and older cultures are/were more focussed on honour, masculine ideas of not saying anything about how you feel, dignity in being silent, etc. This is certainly not to be celebrated; it is simply to point out that there is a bias in the West for mental health research after terrorist attacks.

In short, the study of mental health after terrorism fits cultural fascinations of the West. However, that does not mean the subject is not worthwhile. The study of disaster, as mentioned, is global, and globally people experience trauma and can suffer from PTSD; globally, countries have public health research trying to find who is most at risk, and who should be helped; globally, there are longitudinal studies (in fact, the Bhopal studies in India have gone on for more than 30 years), and there are similar problems overall. Clearly, disasters can have an impact on the mental health of people, and terrorism is no different; disasters are studied worldwide, and terrorism should be no exception simply because of it being mainly a Western study field.

As in all things, science is driven by cultural factors. For example, the Matthew effect, coined by Robert Merton, showcases that *scientific disciplines that receive attention, will get more attention because they receive attention* [125]. Thus, it becomes self-enhancing: mental health after terrorism gets studied, which will lead to more studies on this subject, or as the passage in the bible where the name of the effect is derived from says "*For unto every one that hath shall be given, and he shall have abundance: but from him that hath not shall be taken away even that which he hath.*" [126] (Matthew 25:29).

## 1.10 Conclusion

Perhaps surprisingly, this chapter's main topic was "uncertainty." Uncertainty on what terrorism is, on how to measure mental disorders, and even uncertainty about the results even of studies on mental health. In addition to that uncertainty (and critique), the central concepts of this book were introduced. Several concepts are a better fit for their own dedicated chapter (e.g. resilience, post-traumatic growth and social support), but the main and most important concepts that will be repeated many times throughout are found here.

Finally, an overview was made of what terrorism studies typically are. They are mainly Western focussed quantitative studies, using self-reported screening scales, focussing on poorly measured PTSD outcomes.

## References


1. Cabaj JL, Musto R, Ghali WA. Public health: who, what, and why? Can J Public Health. 2019;110:340–3.
2. Namey EE, Guest G. Public health research methods. SAGE publishers; 2014.
3. Valles S. Philosophy of population health: philosophy for a new public health era. London: Routledge; 2018.
4. Baldwin L, Fleming ML. Introduction to public health. Elsevier; 2008.
5. Lindert J, Bilsen J, Jakubauskiene M. Public mental health. Eur J Pub Health. 2017;27:32–5.
6. Patel V, Prince M. Global mental health. JAMA. 2010;303:1976.
7. Prince M, Patel V, Saxena S, et al. No health without mental health. Lancet. 2007;370:859–77.
8. Quarantelli EL. DISASTER CRISIS MANAGEMENT: A SUMMARY OF RESEARCH FINDINGS. J Manag Stud. 1988;25:373–85.
9. Makwana N. Disaster and its impact on mental health: a narrative review. J Family Med Prim Care. 2019;8:3090.
10. Neria Y, Nandi A, Galea S. Post-traumatic stress disorder following disasters: a systematic review. Psychol Med. 2008;38:467–80.
11. Weisaeth L. The European history of psychotraumatology. J Trauma Stress. 15.
12. Ursano RJ, Fullerton CS, Weisaeth L, et al. Textbook of disaster psychiatry. Cambridge; 2017.
13. Zibulewsky J. Defining disaster: the emergency department perspective. Baylor Univ Med Cent Proc. 2001;14:144–9.
14. Hartman CW, Squires GD. There is no such thing as a natural disaster: race, class, and Hurricane Katrina. Routledge; 2006.
15. Dückers M, Frerks G, Birkmann J. Exploring the plexus of context and consequences: an empirical test of a theory of disaster vulnerability. Int J Disas Risk Reduct. 2015;13:85–95.
16. Herman J. Trauma and recovery. New York: Basic Books; 1992.
17. Alex C. The definition of terrorism: a report. Stationery Office; 2007.
18. DUYVESTEYN I. How new is the new terrorism? Stud Conflict Terrorism. 2004;27:439–54.
19. UNODC. Defining terrorism. United Nations. 2018. https://www.unodc.org/e4j/en/terrorism/module-4/key-issues/defining-terrorism.html. Accessed 17 Jan 2026.
20. Shanahan T. Defining terrorism. In: Handbook of critical terrorism studies. New York: Routledge; 2016.
21. Greene A. DEFINING TERRORISM: ONE SIZE FITS ALL? Int Compar Law Quart. 2017;66:411–40.
22. Schmid AP. Defining terrorism 2023.
23. Rapoport DC. The four waves of rebel terror and September 11. 2002.
24. FBI. §2331. Definitions. 2009. https://www.govinfo.gov/content/pkg/USCODE-2009-title18/html/USCODE-2009-title18-partI-chap113B-sec2331.htm. Accessed 17 Jan 2026.
25. George B, Howard R. Principles of human knowledge and Three dialogues. Oxford University Press; 2009.
26. Edwards DS, McMenemy L, Stapley SA, et al. 40 years of terrorist bombings – a meta-analysis of the casualty and injury profile. Injury. 2016;47:646–52.
27. Almogy G, Rivkind AI. Terror in the 21st century: milestones and prospects—Part I. Curr Probl Surg. 2007;44:496–554.
28. James B. A line in the sand: Britain, France and the struggle for the mastery of the Middle East. Simon & Schuster; 2012.
29. Lawrence W. The looming tower: Al-Qaeda's road to 9/11. Penguin Books; 2011.
30. Robin W. Dreams and shadows: the future of the middle east. Penguin Books; 2014.
31. Durodié B, Wainwright D. Terrorism and post-traumatic stress disorder: a historical review. Lancet Psychiatry. 2019;6:61–71.
32. Verger P, Dab W, Lamping DL, et al. The psychological impact of terrorism: an epidemiologic study of posttraumatic stress disorder and associated factors in victims of the 1995–1996 bombings in France. Am J Psychiatry. 2004;161:1384–9.

33. American Psychiatric Association. Diagnostic and Statistical Manual of Mental Disorders. 5th ed. American Psychiatric Association. 2013. Epub ahead of print 22 May 2013. https://doi.org/10.1176/appi.books.9780890425596.
34. Van Overmeire R. The association between exposure to terrorist attacks and mental health in Belgium. Thesis, Vrije Universiteit Brussel, 2021.
35. World Health Organization. Mental health. 2026. https://www.who.int/health-topics/mental-health#tab=tab_1. Accessed 18 Jan 2026.
36. Satcher D, Friel S, Bell R. Natural and manmade disasters and mental health. JAMA. 2007;298:2540.
37. World Health Organization. ICD-11: International classification of diseases. 11th ed. 2022.
38. Arias D, Saxena S, Verguet S. Quantifying the global burden of mental disorders and their economic value. EClin Med. 2022;54:101675.
39. Chan JKN, Solmi M, Lo HKY, et al. All-cause and cause-specific mortality in people with depression: a large-scale systematic review and meta-analysis of relative risk and aggravating or attenuating factors, including antidepressant treatment. World Psychiatry. 2025;24:404–21.
40. Meng R, Yu C, Liu N, et al. Association of depression with all-cause and cardiovascular disease mortality among adults in China. JAMA Netw Open. 2020;3:e1921043.
41. Ford E, Clark C, McManus S, et al. Common mental disorders, unemployment and welfare benefits in England. Public Health. 2010;124:675–81.
42. Pandarakalam JP. CHALLENGES OF TREATMENT-RESISTANT DEPRESSION. Psychiatr Danub. 2018;30:273–84.
43. Telesia L, Kaushik A, Kyriakopoulos M. The role of stigma in children and adolescents with mental health difficulties. Curr Opin Psychiatry. 2020;33:571–6.
44. DePierro J, Lowe SM, Haugen PT, et al. Mental health stigma and barriers to care in World Trade Center responders: results from a large, population-based health monitoring cohort. Am J Ind Med. 2021;64:208–16.
45. Mascayano F, Armijo JE, Yang LH. Addressing stigma relating to mental illness in low- and middle-income countries. Front Psychiatry; 6. Epub ahead of print 11 March 2015. https://doi.org/10.3389/fpsyt.2015.00038.
46. Rossa-Roccor V, Schmid P, Steinert T. Victimization of people with severe mental illness outside and within the mental health care system: results on prevalence and risk factors from a multicenter study. Front Psychiatry; 11. Epub ahead of print 8 September 2020. https://doi.org/10.3389/fpsyt.2020.563860.
47. Løvstad M, Månum G, Wisløff-Aase K, et al. Persons injured in the 2011 terror attacks in Norway – relationship between post-traumatic stress symptoms, emotional distress, fatigue, sleep, and pain outcomes, and medical and psychosocial factors. Disabil Rehabil. 2020;42:3126–34.
48. Van Overmeire R, Muysewinkel E, Van Keer R-L, et al. Victims of the terrorist attacks in Belgium and professional mental health aid barriers: a qualitative study. Front Psychiatry; 12. Epub ahead of print 2 July 2021. https://doi.org/10.3389/fpsyt.2021.638272.
49. Tucker P, Pfefferbaum B, Watson K, et al. Problems and needs persist for Oklahoma city bombing survivors many years later. Behav Sci. 2021;11:19.
50. Lynch O, Argomaniz J. Victims of terrorism and political violence: identity, needs, and service delivery in Northern Ireland and Great Britain. Terror Polit Violence. 2017;29:464–82.
51. Brodie B. Lectures illustrative of certain local nervous affections. London: A. Spottiswoode; 1837.
52. Mayo T. Medical testimony and evidence in cases of lunacy: being the Croonian lectures delivered before the Royal College of Physicians in 1853; with an essay on the Conditions of Mental Soundness. Michigan: J. W. Parker and son; 1854.
53. Andrew S. Desperate remedies: psychiatry and the mysteries of mental illness. Allen Lane; 2022.
54. Horwitz AVV. PTSD: a short history. Johns Hopkins University Press; 2018.
55. Sadowsky JHal. The empire of depression: a new history. Polity Press; 2021.

56. Zhang Z, Zhang L, Zhang G, et al. The effect of CBT and its modifications for relapse prevention in major depressive disorder: a systematic review and meta-analysis. BMC Psychiatry. 2018;18:50.
57. Zhang Y, Li Z, Feng Q, et al. Global, regional and national burdens of major depression disorders and its attributable risk factors in adolescents and young adults aged 10–24 years from 1990 to 2021. BMC Psychiatry. 2025;25:399.
58. World Health Organization. Depressive disorder (depression). 2025. https://www.who.int/news-room/fact-sheets/detail/depression. Accessed 18 Jan 2026.
59. Haroz EE, Ritchey M, Bass JK, et al. How is depression experienced around the world? A systematic review of qualitative literature. Soc Sci Med. 2017;183:151–62.
60. American Psychiatric Association. Diagnostic and statistical manual of mental disorders. American Psychiatric Association Publishing, 2022. Epub ahead of print 18 March 2022. https://doi.org/10.1176/appi.books.9780890425787.
61. Paris J. The mistreatment of major depressive disorder. Can J Psychiatry. 2014;59:148–51.
62. Zimmerman M, Ellison W, Young D, et al. How many different ways do patients meet the diagnostic criteria for major depressive disorder? Compr Psychiatry. 2015;56:29–34.
63. Meier SM, Deckert J. Genetics of anxiety disorders. Curr Psychiatry Rep. 2019;21:16.
64. Bandelow B, Michaelis S. Epidemiology of anxiety disorders in the 21st century. Dialogues Clin Neurosci. 2015;17:327–35.
65. Maron E, Nutt D. Biological markers of generalized anxiety disorder. Dialogues Clin Neurosci. 2017;19:147–58.
66. American Psychiatric Association. Diagnostic and statistical manual of mental disorders. 4th ed. 1994.
67. Gros DF, Price M, Magruder KM, et al. Symptom overlap in posttraumatic stress disorder and major depression. Psychiatry Res. 2012;196:267–70.
68. GeorgeA B. The end of trauma. New York: Basic Books; 2021.
69. Michalopoulos LM, Meinhart M, Yung J, et al. Global posttrauma symptoms: a systematic review of qualitative literature. Trauma Violence Abuse. 2020;21:406–20.
70. Friedman MJ. PTSD history and overview. PTSD: National Center for PTSD. 2014. https://www.ptsd.va.gov/professional/treat/essentials/history_ptsd.asp. Accessed 15 Feb 2026.
71. Chicco M, Tebala GD. War trauma in Homer's Iliad: a trauma registry perspective. Eur J Trauma Emerg Surg. 2021;47:773–8.
72. Van Lommel K. The recognition of roman soldiers' mental impairment. Acta Cl; 56.
73. Melchior AA. Caesar in Vietnam: did Roman soldiers suffer from post-traumatic stress disorder? Greece and Rome; 58.
74. Page H. Injuries of the spine and spinal cord without apparent mechanical lesion, and nervous shock: in their surgical and medico-legal aspects. London: J&A Churchill; 1883.
75. Peter L. Shell shock: traumatic neurosis and the British soldiers of the First World War. Palgrave; 2002.
76. Harrington R. On the tracks of trauma: railway spine reconsidered. Social Hist Med. 2003;16:209–23.
77. Freud S. The aetiology of hysteria. Standard Edition. London: Hogarth Press, 1896.
78. Jung C. De scheppende mens: over het fenomeen van de geest in kunst en wetenschap. Lemniscaat Modern Antiquariaat; 2000.
79. Tuchman BW. The guns of August: the classic bestselling account of the outbreak of the First World War. Penguin Books; 2014.
80. Adams MCC. Living hell: the dark side of the Civil War. The Johns Hopkins University Press; 2014.
81. Pai A, Suris A, North C. Posttraumatic stress disorder in the DSM-5: controversy, change, and conceptual considerations. Behav Sci. 2017;7:7.
82. Friedman MJ, Resick PA, Keane TM. PTSD from DSM-III to DSM-5. In: Friedman MJ, Keane TM, Resick PA, editors. Handbook of PTSD. New York: Guilford Press; 2014.
83. McNally RJ. Can we fix PTSD in DSM-V? Depress Anxiety. 2009;26:597–600.

84. Muysewinkel E, Stene LE, Van Deynse H, et al. Post-what stress? A review of methods of research on posttraumatic stress during COVID-19. J Anxiety Disord. 2024;102:102829.
85. Asmundson GJG, Taylor S. Garbage in, garbage out: the tenuous state of research on PTSD in the context of the COVID-19 pandemic and infodemic. J Anxiety Disord. 2021;78:102368.
86. Ishtiaq H, Batool TE, Mamoon B, et al. Mental health problems in Pakistani society as a consequence of violence and trauma: a case for better integration of care. Cureus. 2025;17:e83486.
87. Potter C, Feeney J, Fowler E, et al. Post-traumatic stress disorder and memory function in older adults exposed to civilian conflict: findings from the Northern Ireland Cohort for the Longitudinal Study of Ageing (NICOLA). Soc Sci Med. 2026;389:118840.
88. Motreff Y, Baubet T, Pirard P, et al. Factors associated with PTSD and partial PTSD among first responders following the Paris terror attacks in November 2015. J Psychiatr Res. 2020;121:143–50.
89. McLaughlin KA, Koenen KC, Friedman MJ, et al. Subthreshold posttraumatic stress disorder in the World Health Organization World Mental Health Surveys. Biol Psychiatry. 2015;77:375–84.
90. Creswell JW. Research design: qualitative, quantitative, and mixed methods approaches. Sage, 2009.
91. Galea S, Ahern J, Resnick H, et al. Psychological sequelae of the September 11 terrorist attacks in New York City. N Engl J Med. 2002;346:982–7.
92. Willig C. Interpretation and analysis. In: Flick U, editor. The Sage handbook of qualitative data analysis. Sage; 2014.
93. Van Overmeire R, Vesentini L, Van Keer R-L, et al. Working experiences of airport employees after a terrorist attack in Belgium: a qualitative study. Int J Disaster Risk Reduct. 2021;64:102515.
94. Van Overmeire R, Van Keer R, Bilsen J. Impact of terrorist attacks on social relationships. Clin Psychol Psychother. 2021;28:1472–81.
95. Stratton SJ. Likert data. Prehosp Disaster Med. 2018;33:117–8.
96. Wesemann U, Applewhite B, Himmerich H. Investigating the impact of terrorist attacks on the mental health of emergency responders: systematic review. BJPsych Open. 2022;8:e107.
97. Zimmerman M. The value and limitations of self-administered questionnaires in clinical practice and epidemiological studies. World Psychiatry. 2024;23:210–2.
98. Eaton WW, Neufeld K, Chen L-S, et al. A comparison of self-report and clinical diagnostic interviews for depression. Arch Gen Psychiatry. 2000;57:217.
99. Kvig EI, Nilssen S. Does method matter? Assessing the validity and clinical utility of structured diagnostic interviews among a clinical sample of first-admitted patients with psychosis: a replication study. Front Psychiatry; 14. Epub ahead of print 3 April 2023. https://doi.org/10.3389/fpsyt.2023.1076299.
100. Martin J, Streit F, Treutlein J, et al. Expert and self-assessment of lifetime symptoms and diagnosis of major depressive disorder in large-scale genetic studies in the general population. Psychiatr Genet. 2017;27:187–96.
101. Head J, Stansfeld SA, Ebmeier KP, et al. Use of self-administered instruments to assess psychiatric disorders in older people: validity of the General Health Questionnaire, the Center for Epidemiologic Studies Depression Scale and the self-completion version of the revised Clinical Interview Schedule. Psychol Med. 2013;43:2649–56.
102. Hoffmann MS, Pine DS, Georgiades K, et al. Comparing mental health semi-structured diagnostic interviews and symptom checklists to predict poor life outcomes: an 8-year cohort study from childhood to young adulthood in Brazil. Lancet Glob Health. 2024;12:e79–89.
103. Hopwood CJ, Morey LC, Edelen MO, et al. A comparison of interview and self-report methods for the assessment of borderline personality disorder criteria. Psychol Assess. 2008;20:81–5.
104. Samuel DB, Hopwood CJ, Ansell EB, et al. Comparing the temporal stability of self-report and interview assessed personality disorder. J Abnorm Psychol. 2011;120:670–80.
105. Van Overmeire R. The myth of psychological debriefings during the corona pandemic. J Glob Health; 10. Epub ahead of print December 2020. https://doi.org/10.7189/jogh.10.020344.

106. Hobfoll SE, Canetti-Nisim D, Johnson RJ, et al. The association of exposure, risk, and resiliency factors with PTSD among Jews and Arabs exposed to repeated acts of terrorism in Israel. J Trauma Stress. 2008;21:9–21.
107. Hoffman YSG, Diamond GM, Lipsitz JD. The challenge of estimating PTSD prevalence in the context of ongoing trauma: the example of Israel during the Second Intifada. J Anxiety Disord. 2011;25:788–93.
108. Silove D, Bateman CR, Brooks RT, et al. Estimating clinically relevant mental disorders in a rural and an urban setting in postconflict Timor Leste. Arch Gen Psychiatry. 2008;65:1205.
109. Steel Z, Chey T, Silove D, et al. Association of torture and other potentially traumatic events with mental health outcomes among populations exposed to mass conflict and displacement. JAMA. 2009;302:537.
110. Bo H-X, Li W, Yang Y, et al. Posttraumatic stress symptoms and attitude toward crisis mental health services among clinically stable patients with COVID-19 in China. Psychol Med. 2021;51:1052–3.
111. Schuurman B. Research on terrorism, 2007–2016: a review of data, methods, and authorship. Terror Polit Violence. 2020;32:1011–26.
112. Razik S, Ehring T, Emmelkamp PMG. Psychological consequences of terrorist attacks: prevalence and predictors of mental health problems in Pakistani emergency responders. Psychiatry Res. 2013;207:80–5.
113. Eşsizoğlu A, Altınöz AE, Sonkurt HO, et al. The risk factors of possible PTSD in individuals exposed to a suicide attack in Turkey. Psychiatry Res. 2017;253:274–80.
114. Yilmaz E, Tamam L, Cengisiz C. Post-traumatic stress disorder among long-term resettled Syrian refugees in Turkey: a comprehensive analysis of pre- and post-migratory factors. Front Psychiatry. 2024;15:1352288.
115. Çınaroğlu M, Yılmazer E, Noyan Ahlatcıoğlu E, et al. Psychological impact of the 2023 Kahramanmaraş earthquakes: a systematic review and meta-analysis of PTSD, depression, and anxiety among Turkish adults Front Public Health; 13 Epub ahead of print 26 August 2025. https://doi.org/10.3389/fpubh.2025.1664212.
116. Fan X, Ning K, Ma TSW, et al. Post-traumatic stress, depression, and anxiety during the 2021 Myanmar conflict: a nationwide population-based survey. Lancet Reg Health Southeast Asia. 2024;26:100396.
117. Seino K, Takano T, Mashal T, et al. Prevalence of and factors influencing posttraumatic stress disorder among mothers of children under five in Kabul, Afghanistan, after decades of armed conflicts. Health Qual Life Outcomes. 2008;6:29.
118. Tinsae T, Shumet S, Tadesse G, et al. Post-traumatic stress disorder in the Ethiopian population dwelling in war-affected communities: a systematic review and meta-analysis. Front Psychiatry. 2024;15:1399013.
119. Ulrich B. Risk society: towards a new modernity. Sage; 2010.
120. Dückers MLA, Alisic E, Brewin CR. A vulnerability paradox in the cross-national prevalence of post-traumatic stress disorder. Br J Psychiatry. 2016;209:300–5.
121. Dückers MLA, Reifels L, De Beurs DP, et al. The vulnerability paradox in global mental health and its applicability to suicide. Br J Psychiatry. 2019:1–6.
122. Peter C. The medicalization of society: on the transformation of human conditions into treatable disorders. Johns Hopkins University Press; 2007.
123. Horwitz AV, Wakefield JC. The loss of sadness: how psychiatry transformed normal sorrow into depressive disorder. Oxford University Press; 2007.
124. Campbell B, Manning J. The rise of victimhood culture. Cham: Springer International Publishing, 2018. Epub ahead of print 2018. https://doi.org/10.1007/978-3-319-70329-9.
125. Merton RK. The Matthew Effect in science. Science (1979). 1968;159:56–63.
126. King James Bible. Bible. 1769.

# Chapter 2
# Surviving Terrorism: Mental Health Issues Among Directly Exposed People

## 2.1 Introduction

This chapter will provide first a general overview of mental health issues present among directly exposed people. Directly exposed people are those who witness the terrorist attack, or are injured by it, or are bereaved because of the attack. That is a very diverse group of people, and to ensure a more thorough understanding, this chapter is divided into certain subsections.

To start with, a general overview of consequences will be given of terrorism on mental health among directly exposed people, as well as the specific groups with a higher risk.

Following this, while the relation between mental health and terrorism is consistent across all countries, methodologies and socio-political situations that may influence mental health impact vary [1–3]. As such, there will be a section on specific attacks, including 9/11, the attack in Oslo, and a general overview of terrorist threat in Israel. This is important to look deeper into specific contexts, to give findings and numbers that can be reasonably compared with each other.

After this, a specific view will be given on specific groups, such as employees returning to work after an attack, or parents and children.

To end this chapter, the difficult task of providing a summary of decades of research lies ahead.

The reader should also be aware that while many terrorist attacks are mentioned, they are often not described in terms of the actual attack. For reference, the reader can find a list of terrorist attacks in the Appendix that describes in short the nature of the attack.



R. Van Overmeire, *Terrorism, Mental Health and Aftercare*,
https://doi.org/10.1007/978-3-032-31560-1_2

## 2.2 Two Main Conclusions of Research

Terrorism exposure is linked with a wide range of mental health problems, with the most common issues being post-traumatic stress disorder (PTSD), depression, and anxiety [4–9]. It is difficult to provide a specific percentage of how many people develop severe issues, as these are very much dependent on context and time.

However, all research points to two main points.

1. A minority develops mental health disorders

Reviews estimate that the percentage of survivors that develop PTSD is around 30–40% [10, 11]. This certainly depends on case to case, however. For example, after 9/11, PTSD percentages in New York varied, but never went above 50%—in fact, they were closer to 20% [12, 13]. The same goes for attacks such as the Paris attacks of 2015, where half a year after the attacks, 18% of survivors reported PTSD [14]. These percentages are even, probably, overestimations compared to clinical interviews, as it is known that self-reported outcomes (which the majority of research in this field is) tend to yield more mental health issues than clinical interviews [15]. Thus, a minority develops mental health issues.

2. However, at the same time, that minority that develops mental health issues tends to have these problems for a long time.

Based on long-term studies, survivors who developed PTSD or other mental health disorders tend to have these problems for a long time. Both for 9/11 as well as the Oklahoma City Bombing, while a minority develops mental health issues, these can still be noticed among this majority of the minority more than decades later [16–19]. For example, even 10–11 years after 9/11, 15.2% still reported PTSD [20].

## 2.3 Which Groups Are Most at Risk?

There are certain groups that research shows are at higher risk of developing mental health issues.

1. Injured survivors

In general, mental health issues and injury are linked, and there are more mental health issues among those who are injured than among those who are not injured, on average [21–23]. For example, a study in Israel shows that more than half of injured survivors of a suicide bombing have PTSD [24].

PTSD adds more burden to people who are injured [25–27]. Especially among those with a TBI, the burden is not just due to the injury, but also due to the long-term care, pressure on family members, etc [25, 28].

A study after the Mumbai attacks in India showed that especially among injured people, mental health issues were severe [29], as well youth who were injured after the attacks in Utøya [27].

Other somatic problems can also be linked with mental health. For example, after 9/11, asthma and PTSD were linked among 9/11 survivors [30].

2. Gender

The role of gender or sex is complex. Overall, across all disasters and trauma, women have more PTSD than men [31, 32]. For example, after the 2003 Istanbul attack, women had a higher chance of developing PTSD and depression than men [33]. There are many different reasons why this might be. Women might experience trauma overall at a younger age. For example, sexual assault. Might experience more trauma overall. It might be that there is a stronger perception of threat. Additionally, less social support, and possibly gender specific psychobiological reactions to trauma [31]. Other studies point out that gender has no direct relation with PTSD, but an indirect one, where women have more PTSD in general because of fear reactions. So, in general, women have more fear, but it is the fear that is linked with more PTSD, not gender directly [34].

3. Minorities

Minorities have more mental health issues after attacks than the majority group [6, 35]. There are several explanations for this. First, it seems that minority groups already have more mental health problems as baseline, due to for example previous trauma exposure [36, 37]. Second, access to mental health care is more difficult due to limited resources and stigma [27, 38–40]. Third, stigmatization in general also plays a role, as for example Muslim Americans were targeted due to the perpetrators being Muslims [37, 41].

4. Those with low social support

Social support leads to lower levels of PTSD [42]. Interestingly, this is a two-way relation. Indeed, people with low social support had more PTSD, but the PTSD itself also affects the way one experiences and views social support. Not surprisingly, survivors had the least social connections and the fewest social relations when they had the most PTSD [43]. There is indeed more pressure on social relationships, for example between spouses, when one suffers from PTSD [44, 45].

Related to this, the occurrence of an attack can also mean that survivors need to reevaluate aspects of their lives. Terrorism and mental health issues can affect the social roles of survivors, the idea of self-control and agency and other parts of the personality, but also how other people related to the survivors [45, 46]. For example, in one study, a mother wanted to ignore the symptoms she was experiencing as this affected her role of being a mother, and being a breadwinner, while others needed to find new friends since they felt misunderstood by their old friends [45]. In general, exposure to terrorism depletes psychosocial resources, due to the overburdening of the social support with stories of the attacks, due to the mental health issues of the survivor pushing people away (e.g. anger issues are much more common among survivors with mental health issues), or due to other factors, such as the social support experiencing problems of their own [45, 47, 48].

Social support and quality of relations important, and disruptions of those social relations was linked to more mental health issues after the Manchester attacks [49]. Four to 6 weeks after—majority of Museum workers after the Tunesia attack of 2015 had mental health issues, mainly in relation to low social support [50], while survivors of the 2002 Bali bombing who had mental health problems were more against social support initiatives [51]. As it is clear that social support is an important, but very complex factor, it will be discussed in a separate chapter.

5. Previous trauma

As mentioned, women and minorities often have more trauma exposure even before exposure to a terrorist attack. It is such previous trauma exposure that is also one of the predictors of PTSD after terrorist attacks [6, 52].

6. Children and adolescents

Children and adolescents are at high risk of developing a multitude of problems. For example, in one study after 9/11, roughly one in ten of minors living in Manhattan developed panic attacks and PTSD-like symptoms [53], while 9% of minors in New York were hospitalized for mental health issues [54].

Children and adolescents directly exposed suffer from, aside from mental health issues, from several other consequences of their exposure. For example, they tend to have worse school performances, and are delayed in finishing schools, which is especially the case among younger children [55, 56].

Children and adolescents also suffer from behavioral problems, in some cases agoraphobia, and substance abuse issues [57–59]. Behavioral problems were in some children linked with respiratory problems, due to dust cloud exposure, but also having a low-income [59, 60]. Substance abuse increased among French exposed adolescents after the London attacks, and increased more than 5–19 times among adolescents exposed to the 9/11 attacks [61, 62].

In addition, a special group are directly exposed children and/or parents. They are very much linked, as children might for example be influenced by the direct exposure of their parents [56], while children who experience severe mental health issues also create mental health issues in their parents [63]. They are also linked by social factors. For example, findings from the Norwegian attacks show that a third of the parents who lost their child lost their job are unable to work and suffer from psychosocial impairment, even up to 8 years after the attack, which in turn affects their other children [64, 65].

Other examples are seen after 9/11 or after the Kenyan bombing, where the depression of mother's was linked with behavioral problems in pre-school children [66, 67]. This relation could even be noted 3 years after 9/11 [68]. Children of rescue workers who intervened during and after 9/11 had more problems than other groups of children [69]. Children, influenced by their parents' exposure, can have lower grades [56].

Children of non-traditional rescue workers (e.g. construction workers) had more issues than traditional rescue workers (e.g. police officers) [69, 70]. Another example comes from the Boston Marathon bombing, where children who had relatives who participated in the subsequent manhunt of the perpetrators had five times more PTSD symptoms than children who had not [71].

Parents seeking out mental health aid for their children were often motivated not by their mental health symptoms, but by their exposure [72].

## 2.4 Mental Health and Specific Terrorist Attacks

One study indicated that PTSD is worse among terrorism survivors than other forms of trauma, while others state that it is roughly the same effect [5]. It seems that it is difficult to make any such grand generalizations due to many different factors. Aside from all factors related to the terrorist attack (e.g. size of the attack, timing, who is targeted, etc), there are two factors that also play a role in the following findings.

First, while survivors might have experienced a terrorist attack, very few studies take into account that what they see as their worst traumatic event (and thus, in diagnostical sense, the cause of their PTSD) is not always terrorism. Studies in Pakistan showed that domestic abuse was a more frequently trauma than terrorism [73], while only 60% of civilians in Northern Ireland exposed to terrorist attacks in answering the PTSD scales [74]. In short, survivors of terrorism might develop PTSD and depression and anxiety, and this can be *associated* with terrorist attacks, but can seldom be said to have been *caused* by terrorist attacks in a scientific way. While it already is methodologically challenging to show the link between exposure and mental health issues, it is made more difficult by the fact that hardly any studies take into account the fact the prior trauma might be the cause of symptoms, and not a risk factor for terrorism-related mental health issues.

Second, an additional and related factor, is that trauma exposure and PTSD rates can differ significantly depending on the country. Countries such as Poland or Ireland have much higher rates than the average European country [75, 76]. Thus, in this section, several terrorist attacks will be viewed within their own context.

### *2.4.1 9/11*

The majority of studies on the relationship between mental health and terrorism among those directly exposed stem from studies after 9/11. As in most social sciences, the biggest event draws the most attention of studies, but at the same time might skew any attempt at generalizing results. However, mental health reactions to 9/11, despite its grand political consequences, are similar to other attacks. For example, after a series of sniper attacks in Washington D.C., acute stress rates were quite similar to those after 9/11 [77].

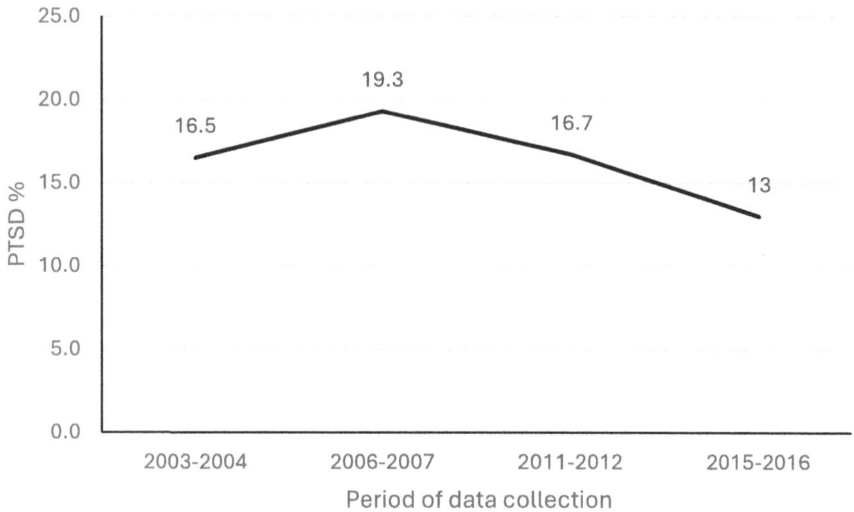


**Fig. 2.1** PTSD percentage among tower-survivors, based on Adams, et al. [9] (Used with permission of the American Psychological Association, from *PTSD and comorbid depression: Social support and self-efficacy in World Trade Center tower survivors 14–15 years after 9/11*, Adams, S.W., et al., Vol. 11(2), 2019; permission conveyed through Copyright Clearance Center, Inc.)

In a similar way to the Oklahoma City Bombing, 9/11 offers a well performed longitudinal analysis. Most interesting, however, is the insight it gives in the short-term aftermath. For example, the weeks after the attacks. From these studies we see that in 5–8 weeks after the attacks, 8.8% of the population had PTSD [12], with as main predictors being gender (women have more PTSD), life stressors in previous 12 months and social support (with low social support predicting PTSD) [12, 78]. Another study showed that the PTSD rates declined from 7.5% in the first month to 0.6% after 6 months, where mainly those directly exposed still experienced PTSD symptoms [13, 79].

Other studies show that in the years following the attacks, PTSD and depression take on unpredictable pathways. As already mentioned by authors about PTSD, symptoms of PTSD will fluctuate [80]. This is notable in Fig. 2.1.

The evolution of PTSD and depression in survivors of 9/11 provides invaluable insight into the progression of mental health issues after terrorist attacks. A longitudinal study of tower survivors shows an increase, and then a slow decrease [9].

**Language and PTSD**

Studies after terrorism also show a link between the words survivors use to describe their trauma and their chance of developing PTSD [81]. One study after 9/11, for example, showed that at a first measurement, survivors who use fewer words referring to the anxiety they experienced had more chance to develop chronic PTSD later on [82].

Women, people with low income, and minorities had an increased chance to develop PTSD and other mental health problems [83]. In addition, there were contextual factors. For example, being on the high floors, being evacuated late, being injured, being caught in the dust cloud, and working for someone who died in the attacks, were all related to higher risk for PTSD [83]. In fact, survivors that were in the towers had much higher risk for substance abuse and PTSD than survivors from surrounding building, even up to 10 years later [84]. Similarly, anxiety symptoms were linked with having someone near the site of the attacks or involved with the rescue effort [85]. Despite the quite consistent high mental health issues, there is little evidence among survivors of an increased risk of suicide [86].

Survivors of terrorist attacks are prone to use alcohol as self-medication. Across all terrorist attacks, 6% of survivors drink more alcohol, and 5.5% develop an alcohol abuse problem [87]. This is equally true for survivors of 9/11, who were noted for having a higher chance to self-medicate. Self-medication through alcohol and binge drinking were common over more than a decade later after the attacks [84, 88–90], which seems to be mainly due to a relation with mental health issues [6, 91]. That does not simply mean that survivors use alcohol as reaction to PTSD, but the reverse also is true: alcohol use makes one more prone to PTSD [39].

Related to this, up to 13 years after 9/11, survivors with mental health issues had more risk of being hospitalized for opioid addiction than those without [92, 93]. This opioid use might be explained from the lack of access to proper healthcare [94]. In fact, it is noticeable that majority people who would seem to have such an addiction, do this to treat cancer-related pain [94]. Others have oversubscribed opioids for 9/11 related rheumatoid arthritis [95]. In fact, only around 6% have no such disease [94]. In addition, it is well documented that opioids were easily prescribed by medical doctors starting around the period of 9/11, with the most famous opioid being OxyContin, which has been related to the later opioid pandemic in the USA [96]. In that sense, the opioid addictions found in the survivors of 9/11 were a symptom of the much broader pandemic.

Other drugs use, such as tobacco and marijuana use, did not increase notably after 9/11. In fact, the increase that was found, stabilized after 3 years [97].

### 2.4.2 Oklahoma City Bombing

Though this chapter aims to provide variation in location and disasters, the purpose of showcasing the Oklahoma City Bombing chapter here in addition to 9/11 is to provide another overview of longitudinal mental health issues among survivors. Studies on survivors are, to the author's knowledge, the longest running surveys in terrorism research, and thus provide invaluable knowledge. A half year after the disaster, roughly 34% of survivors had PTSD [16]. Seven years later, this was 26% [98]. However, 25 years later, this rose to 37% [99]. Why this might be, is somewhat unclear. Indeed, needs are persistent with the survivors, including healthcare and financial needs [100], but it might be that in 25 years, there were indeed other traumatic events that happened. This is not unreasonable, considering that 70% of the world population is exposed to trauma at some point in their lives [101, 102].

### 2.4.3 Oslo

In general, Oslo studies show that greater exposure, being female, being a migrant, and having low social support is related to more mental health issues [27, 42, 103]. In the first half year after the attack, the PTSD rates of survivors were six times higher than the general population [104]. This PTSD was often linked with shame and guilt as well [105]. In the long term, it seems that PTSD is quite stable, meaning, that even up to 8 years after the attacks, specific mental health issues do not increase, but also do not decrease [106].

Related to this stability of PTSD, survivors still experienced trauma reminders (e.g. intrusive thoughts or memories of the attacks) 8½ years after the attacks [107, 108]. Furthermore, 90% of all survivors had at least one trauma reminder in the past month in one study, and around a third very often, which impacts their social functioning [107]. In the long term, mainly auditory reminders of the attack, but the reminders fluctuate, as well as their severity for the PTSD [109]. Half of the survivors still had insomnia symptoms years later, and even siblings and parents suffered from insomnia and fatigue [110–112].

The consequences are also seen in other areas of the survivors' lives, such as their coping skills. Survivors with PTSD tended to have maladaptive appraisals [106]. These are appraisals such as "Nothing good ever happens to me," "I will never be the same person again," and "I should have coped better" are linked with PTSD [113]. Half of the survivors also experienced strong distrust and fear for others; not only of the perpetrator, but even people trying to help them, such as medical personnel [114]. However, there was quite a lot of trust in the justice system in both survivors and parents, which even increased in the long term [115].

Other problems that occur among survivors are migraines. In the first half year, there was significant increase of migraines among survivors, higher than the national average [116]. While this might be due to stress, the link between migraines and stress remains unclear [117], though there is some evidence that somatic symptoms such as headaches are predictors for PTSD [118].

The parents of deceased children also suffer from severe emotional reactions and PTSD [119]. Parents of deceased children had three times more PTSD and five times more anxiety than the general population [120].

Yet, among the majority of survivors there was also evidence of posttraumatic growth, indicating a new appreciation of parts of life and others [121]. In fact, there was also evidence that visiting the site attack could be beneficial [122].

### 2.4.4 Christchurch Attack

The Christchurch attack is atypical: it was an attack on a minority group. As the previous sections made clear, minority groups experience more mental health issues in general. Aside from the higher rates of PTSD [123], those affected experienced in addition to a higher perception of terrorism [124]. Furthermore, politically their worries became more focused on the process of justice, gun-control laws, etc [125].

However, there was also a feeling of greater community, and in fact, the impact of the attack on the mental health of those affected was not as large as one would expect based on the other attacks in this chapter [124]. Even more so, post-traumatic growth through religious coping was present among directly exposed Muslim. However, this was less so among higher educated Muslims, and those with family tensions [126].

### 2.4.5 Other Attacks

**Northern Ireland**
A study of adolescent survivors after a bombing in Northern Ireland in 1998 showed high PTSD, which was mainly linked with the idea of seeing someone dying, and thinking they themselves were going to die [127]. Interestingly, among residents of the town, visiting the scene of the attack after the attack was also linked with high PTSD rates [128], which is not found in other studies after other attacks [122]. In fact, these were higher rates than those who left the scene of attack just before the attack occurred [128].

**Kenya**
Kenyan survivors of the U.S. embassy bombing in Kenya had very high rates of PTSD (28% 3 years later) and more functioning problems [129]. The ethnic background was sometimes predictive of PTSD, possibly due to social support and stigma in certain ethnicities in Kenya [130]. Among U.S. embassy personnel, 32% had PTSD [131]. In both, few had psychiatric treatment, and being injured in the hospital seemed to have been good in lower depression [129].

**United Kingdom Survivors**
A study of United Kingdom citizens who were survivors of various attacks showed that most screened positive for depressive or anxiety symptoms, and around 15% feeling a risk to their job [132]. This reflects also in that a third of United Kingdom survivors of various terrorist attacks have reduced their working hours, and taken more sick leave [133], indicating the economic stress that mental health issues can bring to survivors.

In addition, one study showed another less obvious consequence of terrorism: the routines that are affected. The London attack of 2005 was an attack on public transport, which for certain survivors of the attacks meant that public transport itself became a struggle [134, 135]. This is something that was also noticed after the sniper attacks in the United States, where walking in the street became a stressor for survivors [136].

**Madrid Attacks**

Studies on the Madrid attacks show a notable decline in PTSD rates. The first month, 35.7% of those affected had PTSD, going to 34.1% after 6 months, and 28.6% after 12 months [137]. People admitted to the emergency room in Madrid after the attacks had high PTSD that did not really change and remained roughly around 40% between the first month and the sixth month [23]. Interestingly, while this was almost half for those injured, this was not even 4% for police officers, for reasons that will be further explored in the next chapter [138]. Among the victims of terrorism in Spain, there was also evidence of post-traumatic growth, most evident among women [139].

**Terrorist Attacks in Turkey, Japan, and Russia**

While hardly studied, research on survivors of the 2003 Istanbul attack in Turkey that 35% had PTSD, and 23% had depression [33], while after the 2015 Ankara attack showed that 24% had PTSD [140, 141]. Also under the radar of the research field is the 1995 Sarin attack. One study showed that roughly 35% of the survivors displayed PTSD, again also showing that being female and being older are risk factors [142, 143]. Important to note is that this study was conducted 5 years after the attacks, yet PTSD was still high [142]. Studies on the Beslan attacks in Russia show that adolescents, and especially boys, are especially affected by distress. After 3 years, there was even an increase in distress in boys [144–148]. Beslan is exceptional in terms of terrorism research in that it is one of the few long-term studies outside what is traditionally seen as the "West."

**Mumbai Terrorist Attacks**

A week after the 2008 Mumbai attacks in India, 30% of the people injured had acute stress disorder diagnosed by a psychiatrist [29, 149]. A follow-up study showed that even 2 years later, more than 60% still showcased distress [150]. Those injured in the attacks had often migrated to Mumbai for work, and were often the breadwinners of their families, and thus were unable to sustain the work they were doing in Mumbai, forcing them to return to their hometowns [150]. As economic studies have shown, the reason for the migration to Mumbai is precisely that the wages there are so much higher than in smaller towns, which is precisely the reason for the mass-migrations to Mumbai [151]. In addition, due to the loss of a family member or the reduced income, other events started occurring, such as children quitting school, or business going bankrupt [150].

### *2.4.6 Israel*

Naturally, the conflict between Palestine and Israel has mental health consequences for all affected, and clearly is related with changing attitudes, behavior, feelings, on both youth and the general population in both Palestine and Isreal [152–156]. In this chapter, Israel is highlighted because there is (1) a wealth of research there that Palestine does not have, (2) it offers a population that is most similar in socio-economic situation to that of other countries in this chapter, making the comparison interesting in the sense that most countries discussed in this book are on population that experience one terrorist attack, while the Israeli population often experienced multiple, and live in a state of continuous threat.

There are indeed indications that the impact of terrorism is different depending on the frequency. Recurrent terrorism might have different effects than single exposure [157]. It has been assumed that this recurrent terrorism would lead to "habituation" in the population. In the case of terrorism, this is when reoccurring threat or attacks do not cause the same reaction, and in fact, people adjust to the constant attacks [158]. This has been important in explaining the lower PTSD rates in the Israeli population. For example, several studies find that find that 9–10% of the people in Israel who experience direct terrorism exposure have PTSD [159–161], while among adolescents one study found that recurrent exposure was associated with around 7% PTSD [162, 163].

However, habituation does not mean that atypically large attacks cannot cause similar reactions as in other countries. For example, after the October 7 attacks in Israel, around 12–15% of the population experienced PTSD in the first half year after the attack [164–167].

Furthermore, the lower impact of terrorism on the mental health in Israel does not mean that the consequences for those who do develop mental health problems is lower. For example, adolescents experience more suicidal ideation and more risk-taking behaviour [162, 168], and there is more substance abuse, such as of tranquilizers and alcohol, among those directly exposed to terrorist attacks [169–171].

There is also a difference between Arab and Jewish Israelis. While the initial impact of terrorism is roughly the same for both groups, Arab Israelis seem to have more mental health issues after terrorist attacks than Jewish Israelis in the long run [165, 172–174]. Arab Israelis, for example, have 2.5 more depression than Jewish Israelis [175].

One of the possible reasons why Arab Israelis might have more issues due to reoccurring terrorism is due to their more limited access to mental health care, due to stigma and limited resources [166]. This is also true for Arab adolescents, who seem to experience more stress than Jewish Israelis, and cope more through anger [176–178].

Another reason is that they are a minority group, which would fit other findings in this chapter where minority groups always have more mental health issues than the majority group. It is important to note that this is not solely because the minority group is Arabic. In fact, one study showed that a minority group within the Jewish Israelis, the Mizrahi group, has more mental health issues due to terrorism and the war in Gaza than the majority group, the Ashkenazi group [179].

**A Short Summary of All Case Studies**

The case studies described provide several insights. First, they show that terrorism affects mental health worldwide, from the USA to Israel to Russia to India to Japan.

Second, they showcase the importance of environmental and contextual factors of an attack, and that having PTSD affects the person on many different levels, such as affecting their opinions, trust and even dreams. In a survivor's daily life, routines might be changed due to the attacks. Financial costs can be high after terrorism, sick leave can become more common, while children might stop going to school and businesses can go bankrupt.

Terrorism also affects communities, and also how these communities function. It can cause rifts in communities, and survivors might be forced to change their entire lives.

## 2.5 Impact on the Workplace

To end the overview of survivors and mental health, a short section on the workplace. After all, terrorist attacks often focus areas that are the workplace of people, and this in itself will also affect the recovery of survivors.

Employees are either present during the attack, or have to return to their workplace after the attacks, wherein the workplace becomes a constant reminder of the attacks. As one survivor of the airport attacks stated:

> This will never be the innocent, safe airport that it once was. That feeling is gone… [180].

Yet, the workplace can also play an important part in a community response to disaster [181].

In general, most employees working in companies affected by terrorism felt a fast return to work was good [180, 182]. However, while employees experienced an initial period of positive reactions, this changed in the long run to impatience [46]. A lack of understanding of the post-terrorism reactions led to changing jobs, bullying, exclusion, etc [45, 46, 180]. Companies needed to be forward looking and needed to seek to make up for lost income, and thus the expectancy was to go to business as usual, which clashed with those survivors for whom the terrorist attacks were central to their experience of work [46, 180]. This creates tension between the personal needs and the workplace needs [183, 184].

Terror exposed employees also felt less safe at the workplace, had a higher perception of terrorist threat, and especially when coupled with mental health issues, tended to view their employer in a more negative daylight [77, 185, 186]. As time passes, there also started to exist a difference between those employees who were "there" and "not there"; as in, those who experienced the attacks and those who did not, as for those exposed, the attacks remain central to their work experience, which creates extra tension on the work floor [180, 187].

The mental health care offered by the company is an important factor. While in all companies there was an offer [180, 181, 188–191], in some cases, the aid offered was deemed insufficient. This due to various reasons, including limited offerings, not feeling understood, and others that are discussed more deeply in a specific chapter on mental health aid [181, 192]. Those who had to seek out extra mental health care outside the company, also had more distress symptoms [193].

Similarly to other groups in this chapter, PTSD and depression were common among employees, and linked with exposure to the terrorist attacks [77, 182, 184, 194–196]. Though, there is a difference of course between directly and indirectly exposed people. For example, while emotional numbness was present among most during the first 10 months [197], directly exposed people were mainly affected by the memory of the attack, which after the memories faded turned into emotional numbing. This emotional numbing was already present in indirectly exposed employees [198].

Not surprisingly, companies that were affected by terrorism had higher sick leave rates and absences, and this especially among those directly exposed to women, and mostly women [199, 200]. This sick leave stabilized after 3 years in Oslo [199], while worker productivity was down a year after 9/11 [201].

**How to Avoid This?**

First, making the workplace into a predictable environment, with a high perception of safety, is important in reducing sickleave [202]. In fact, when there is a high perception of safety, this can decrease sick leave by 30% [203]. Second, social support of colleagues and managers can lower both the PTSD and the sick leave by 20% and decrease mental health issues [204, 205]. Third, employees should avoid having a low sense of control over their work, and have clear roles [200, 206].

In all these factors, the role of the manager is important. A manager who can provide role clarity, avoid conflicts, give appreciation to employees, avoid the sense of "business as usual," and provide predictability in the workplace can ensure lower mental health issues among employees [207–210]. Additionally, they can increase the sense of safety by providing information on evacuation routes.

To end this section, another testimony of an employee and survivor of the airport attack in Belgium that began this section, to showcase the response when there is a perception that nothing changed and nobody listens:

> We're almost three years later, and (the safety situation) only gets worse—"worse" is maybe exaggerated. Okay, there are people (security personnel) everywhere—but they don't do anything. And politics, yeah, the first months you can do everything, but [...]It won't last 5 years or it happens again. We can only tell them (management and politicians) what's happening, but they won't be able to say 'Wir haben das nicht gewust' [180].

## 2.6 Conclusion

Providing a conclusion for decades of research is a challenge. This chapter has attempted to provide the reader key principles of the research, and at the same time showcase that terrorist attacks always have sui generis aspects (e.g. the physical layout of the Twin Towers plays a role in prediction of PTSD). If successful, this chapter should have outlined the diversity in terrorism research on survivors, as well showcasing the difficulties in really pointing to key factors of what is associated with the mental health issues.

In addition, this chapter showed a diversity in focusses of research, with Oslo studies having slightly other elements that are deemed important compared to, for example, the studies on the Mumbai attacks. Overall, however, very few studies actually focus on the impact of terrorism on communities, or even the consequences of terrorism for people other than the survivors or parents of victims. For example, the Mumbai attacks show that indeed, if the breadwinner is hurt, this has severe consequences beyond distress.

This lack of attention for such factors is perhaps due to terrorism studies being mainly Western focused, and thus perhaps more concerned with the individual instead of the community. Either way, the evidence that exists indicates that more attention should be given to broader approaches, taking into account more than PTSD.

## References

1. Laugharne J, Janca A, Widiger T. Posttraumatic stress disorder and terrorism: 5 years after 9/11. Curr Opin Psychiatry. 2007;20:36–41.
2. Verger P, Dab W, Lamping DL, et al. The psychological impact of terrorism: an epidemiologic study of posttraumatic stress disorder and associated factors in victims of the 1995–1996 bombings in France. Am J Psychiatry. 2004;161:1384–9.
3. Abenhaim L, Dab W, Salmi LR. Study of civilian victims of terrorist attacks (FRANCE 1982–1987). J Clin Epidemiol. 1992;45:103–9.
4. Rubacka JM, Schmeidler J, Nomura Y, et al. The relationship between PTSD arousal symptoms and depression among mothers exposed to the World Trade Center attacks. J Nerv Ment Dis. 2008;196:504–7.
5. Pozza A, Bossini L, Ferretti F, et al. The effects of terrorist attacks on symptom clusters of PTSD: a comparison with victims of other traumatic events. Psychiatry Q. 2019;90:587–99.
6. Adams RE, Boscarino JA. Predictors of PTSD and delayed PTSD after disaster. J Nerv Ment Dis. 2006;194:485–93.
7. Boscarino JA, Kirchner HL, Hoffman SN, et al. PTSD and alcohol use after the World Trade Center attacks: a longitudinal study. J Trauma Stress. 2011;24:515–25.
8. Bossini L, Ilaria C, Koukouna D, et al. PTSD in victims of terroristic attacks – a comparison with the impact of other traumatic events on patients' lives. Psychiatr Pol. 2016;50:907–21.
9. Adams SW, Bowler RM, Russell K, et al. PTSD and comorbid depression: social support and self-efficacy in World Trade Center tower survivors 14–15 years after 9/11. Psychol Trauma. 2019;11:156–64.
10. Whalley MG, Brewin CR. Mental health following terrorist attacks. Br J Psychiatry. 2007;190:94–6.
11. Paz García-Vera M, Sanz J, Gutiérrez S. A systematic review of the literature on posttraumatic stress disorder in victims of terrorist attacks. Psychol Rep. 2016;119:328–59.
12. Galea S. Posttraumatic stress disorder in Manhattan, New York City, after the September 11th terrorist attacks. J Urban Health. 2002;79:340–53.
13. Galea S. Trends of probable post-traumatic stress disorder in New York City after the September 11 terrorist attacks. Am J Epidemiol. 2003;158:514–24.

14. Vandentorren S, Pirard P, Sanna A, et al. Healthcare provision and the psychological, somatic and social impact on people involved in the terror attacks in January 2015 in Paris: cohort study. Br J Psychiatry. 2018;212:207–14.
15. Williams R, Bell C, Kaufman KR. The thematic series on the psychosocial and mental health impacts of terrorism and collective violence: narrative review of common themes from diverse events, places and research methods. BJPsych Open. 2025;11:e169.
16. North CS, Pfefferbaum B, Kawasaki A, et al. Psychosocial adjustment of directly exposed survivors 7 years after the Oklahoma City bombing. Compr Psychiatry. 2011;52:1–8.
17. North CS. A longitudinal follow-up study of Oklahoma City bombing survivors in the first quarter century after the disaster. Ann Clin Psychiatry; 35. Epub ahead of print May 2023. https://doi.org/10.12788/acp.0095.
18. Perlman SE, Friedman S, Galea S, et al. Short-term and medium-term health effects of 9/11. Lancet. 2011;378:925–34.
19. Jacobson MH, Norman C, Nguyen A, et al. Longitudinal determinants of depression among World Trade Center Health Registry enrollees, 14–15 years after the 9/11 attacks. J Affect Disord. 2018;229:483–90.
20. Caramanica K, Brackbill RM, Liao T, et al. Comorbidity of 9/11-related PTSD and depression in the World Trade Center Health Registry 10–11 years postdisaster. J Trauma Stress. 2014;27:680–8.
21. Zatzick DF, Jurkovich GJ, Fan M-Y, et al. Association between posttraumatic stress and depressive symptoms and functional outcomes in adolescents followed up longitudinally after injury hospitalization. Arch Pediatr Adolesc Med. 2008;162:642.
22. DF ZATZICK, FP RIVARA, AB NATHENS, et al. A nationwide US study of post-traumatic stress after hospitalization for physical injury. Psychol Med. 2007;37:1469–80.
23. Fraguas D, Terán S, Conejo-Galindo J, et al. Posttraumatic stress disorder in victims of the March 11 attacks in Madrid admitted to a hospital emergency room: 6-month follow-up. Eur Psychiatry. 2006;21:143–51.
24. Shussman N, Mintz A, Zamir G, et al. Posttraumatic stress disorder in hospitalized terrorist bombing attack victims. J Trauma Inj Inf Crit Care. 2011;70:1546–50.
25. Sample PL, Greene D, Johns NR. Life–bombing–injury–life: a qualitative follow-up study of Oklahoma City bombing survivors with TBI. Brain Inj. 2012;26:1670–83.
26. Haagsma JA, Polinder S, Toet H, et al. Beyond the neglect of psychological consequences: post-traumatic stress disorder increases the non-fatal burden of injury by more than 50%. Inj Prev. 2011;17:21–6.
27. Bugge I, Dyb G, Stensland SØ, et al. Physical injury and posttraumatic stress reactions. A study of the survivors of the 2011 shooting massacre on Utøya Island, Norway. J Psychosom Res. 2015;79:384–90.
28. Le Moullec D, Salvadori A, Constantin P, et al. Traumatic brain injury and posttraumatic stress disorder: overlap in underlying substrates. J Trauma Inj Inf Crit Care. 2011;71:1923–4.
29. Joseph J, Jaswal S. Psychosocial framework for understanding psychological distress among survivors of the November 26, 2008 Mumbai terror attack: beyond traumatic experiences and emergency medical care. Prehosp Disaster Med. 2014;29:330–8.
30. Brackbill RM. Asthma and posttraumatic stress symptoms 5 to 6 years following exposure to the World Trade Center terrorist attack. JAMA. 2009;302:502.
31. Olff M, Langeland W, Draijer N, et al. Gender differences in posttraumatic stress disorder. Psychol Bull. 2007;133:183–204.
32. Birkeland MS, Blix I, Solberg Ø, et al. Gender differences in posttraumatic stress symptoms after a terrorist attack: a network approach. Front Psychol; 8. Epub ahead of print 1 December 2017. https://doi.org/10.3389/fpsyg.2017.02091.
33. Zara Page A, Kaplan H, Erdogan N, et al. Posttraumatic stress and depression reactions among survivors of the Istanbul November 2003 terrorist attacks. J Aggress Maltreat Trauma. 2009;18:280–92.
34. Laufer A, Solomon Z. Gender differences in PTSD in Israeli youth exposed to terror attacks. J Interpers Violence. 2009;24:959–76.

35. Adams RE, Boscarino JA, Galea S. Alcohol use, mental health status and psychological well-being 2 years after the World Trade Center attacks in New York City. Am J Drug Alcohol Abuse. 2006;32:203–24.
36. Roberts AL, Gilman SE, Breslau J, et al. Race/ethnic differences in exposure to traumatic events, development of post-traumatic stress disorder, and treatment-seeking for post-traumatic stress disorder in the United States. Psychol Med. 2011;41:71–83.
37. Padela AI, Heisler M. The association of perceived abuse and discrimination after September 11, 2001, with psychological distress, level of happiness, and health status among Arab Americans. Am J Public Health. 2010;100:284–91.
38. Piwowarczyk L, Rous D, Mancuso A, et al. Impact of the Boston marathon bombing and its aftermath on refugees and survivors of torture. J Immigr Minor Health. 2016;18:764–70.
39. Boscarino JA, Adams RE, Figley CR. Mental health service use 1-year after the World Trade Center disaster: implications for mental health care. Gen Hosp Psychiatry. 2004;26:346–58.
40. Bugge I, Dyb G, Stensland SØ, et al. Physical injury and somatic complaints: the mediating role of posttraumatic stress symptoms in young survivors of a terror attack. J Trauma Stress. 2017;30:229–36.
41. Samari, Goleen. Islamophobia and public health in the United States. Am J Public Health. 2016;106:e13.
42. Birkeland MS, Hansen MB, Blix I, et al. For whom does time heal wounds? Individual differences in stability and change in posttraumatic stress after the 2011 Oslo bombing. J Trauma Stress. 2017;30:19–26.
43. Hamwey MK, Pollari CD, Osahan S, et al. Associations of embeddedness and posttraumatic stress disorder among 9/11 survivors. Epidemiologia. 2021;2:608–20.
44. Menendez AM, Molloy J, Magaldi MC. HEALTH RESPONSES OF NEW YORK CITY FIREFIGHTER SPOUSES AND THEIR FAMILIES POST-SEPTEMBER 11, 2001 TERRORIST ATTACKS. Issues Ment Health Nurs. 2006;27:905–17.
45. Van Overmeire R, Van Keer R, Bilsen J. Impact of terrorist attacks on social relationships. Clin Psychol Psychother. 2021;28:1472–81.
46. Stancombe J, Williams R, Drury J, et al. People's experiences of distress and psychosocial care following a terrorist attack: interviews with survivors of the Manchester Arena bombing in 2017. BJPsych Open. 2022;8:e41.
47. Hobfoll SE, Canetti-Nisim D, Johnson RJ. Exposure to terrorism, stress-related mental health symptoms, and defensive coping among Jews and Arabs in Israel. J Consult Clin Psychol. 2006;74:207–18.
48. Tran DV, North CS. The prevalence, characteristics, and correlates of anger among survivors of the 9/11 World Trade Center attacks. Ann Clin Psychiatry. 2017;29:235–41.
49. Stancombe J, Williams R, Drury J, et al. Trajectories of distress and recovery, secondary stressors and social cure processes in people who used the resilience hub after the Manchester Arena bombing. BJPsych Open. 2023;9:e143.
50. Fekih-Romdhane F, Chennoufi L, Cheour M. PTSD and depression among museum workers after the March 18 Bardo Museum terrorist attack. Community Ment Health J. 2017;53:852–8.
51. Stevens GJ, Dunsmore JC, Agho KE, et al. Coping support factors among Australians affected by terrorism: 2002 Bali bombing survivors speak. Med J Aust. 2013;199:772–5.
52. Chemtob CM, Nomura Y, Abramovitz RA. Impact of conjoined exposure to the World Trade Center attacks and to other traumatic events on the behavioral problems of preschool children. Arch Pediatr Adolesc Med. 2008;162:126.
53. Pfefferbaum B, Stuber J, Galea S, et al. Panic reactions to terrorist attacks and probable posttraumatic stress disorder in adolescents. J Trauma Stress. 2006;19:217–28.
54. Gargano LM, Locke SH, Alper HE, et al. Hospitalizations among World Trade Center Health Registry enrollees who were under 18 years of age on 9/11, 2001–2016. Int J Environ Res Public Health. 2021;18:7527.
55. Strøm IF, Dyb G, Wentzel-Larsen T, et al. Terror leaves adolescents behind: identifying risk and protective factors for high-school completion among survivors of terrorism. J Trauma Stress. 2023;36:750–61.

56. Pfefferbaum B, Simic Z, North CS. Parent-reported child reactions to the September 11, 2001 World Trade Center attacks (New York USA) in relation to parent post-disaster psychopathology three years after the event. Prehosp Disaster Med. 2018;33:558–64.
57. Stuber J, Galea S, Pfefferbaum B, et al. Behavior problems in New York City's children after the September 11, 2001, terrorist attacks. Am J Orthopsychiatry. 2005;75:190–200.
58. Hoven CW, Duarte CS, Lucas CP, et al. Psychopathology among New York City Public School children 6 months after September 11. Arch Gen Psychiatry. 2005;62:545.
59. Mann M, Li J, Farfel MR, et al. Adolescent behavior and PTSD 6–7 years after the World Trade Center terrorist attacks of September 11, 2001. Disaster Health. 2014;2:121–9.
60. Stellman SD, Thomas PA, Osahan S, et al. Respiratory health of 985 children exposed to the World Trade Center disaster: report on World Trade Center Health Registry wave 2 follow-up, 2007–2008. J Asthma. 2013;50:354–63.
61. Chemtob CM, Nomura Y, Josephson L, et al. Substance use and functional impairment among adolescents directly exposed to the 2001 World Trade Center attacks. Disasters. 2009;33:337–52.
62. Coulon N, Grenon M, Consigny M, et al. PTSD in French adolescent victims following the London attack in March 2017: data from the first step of the AVAL study. Front Psychiatry; 13 Epub ahead of print 24 February 2022. https://doi.org/10.3389/fpsyt.2022.728133.
63. Kerns CE, Elkins RM, Carpenter AL, et al. Caregiver distress, shared traumatic exposure, and child adjustment among area youth following the 2013 Boston Marathon bombing. J Affect Disord. 2014;167:50–5.
64. Nordström E-EL, Thimm JC, Kaltiala R, et al. Prolonged grief, post-traumatic stress, and functional impairment in parents and siblings 8 years after the 2011 Utøya terror attack. Eur J Psychotraumatol; 13 Epub ahead of print 19 December 2022. https://doi.org/10.1080/20008066.2022.2152930.
65. Thimm JC, Kristensen P, Aulie IF, et al. The associations of grief-related rumination with prolonged grief and posttraumatic stress symptoms: a longitudinal study of bereaved after the 2011 terror attack in Norway. Clin Psychol Psychother; 31. Epub ahead of print 11 January 2024. https://doi.org/10.1002/cpp.2950.
66. Chemtob CM, Nomura Y, Rajendran K, et al. Impact of maternal posttraumatic stress disorder and depression following exposure to the September 11 attacks on preschool children's behavior. Child Dev. 2010;81:1129–41.
67. Pfefferbaum B, North CS, Narayanan P, et al. The relationship between maternal psychopathology and parental perceptions of their children's reactions in survivors of the 1998 US Embassy bombing in Nairobi, Kenya. Ann Clin Psychiatry. 2019;31:260–70.
68. Nomura Y, Chemtob CM. Effect of maternal psychopathology on behavioral problems in preschool children exposed to terrorism. Arch Pediatr Adolesc Med. 2009;163:531.
69. Uchida M, Feng H, Feder A, et al. Parental posttraumatic stress and child behavioral problems in world trade center responders. Am J Ind Med. 2018;61:504–14.
70. Duarte CS, Hoven CW, Wu P, et al. Posttraumatic stress in children with first responders in their families. J Trauma Stress. 2006;19:301–6.
71. Comer JS, Kerns CE, Elkins RM, et al. ADJUSTMENT AMONG CHILDREN WITH RELATIVES WHO PARTICIPATED IN THE MANHUNT FOLLOWING THE BOSTON MARATHON ATTACK. Depress Anxiety. 2014;31:542–50.
72. DeVoe ER, Bannon WM, Klein TP. Post-9/11 helpseeking by New York City parents on behalf of highly exposed young children. Am J Orthopsychiatry. 2006;76:167–75.
73. Ishtiaq H, Batool TE, Mamoon B, et al. Mental health problems in Pakistani society as a consequence of violence and trauma: a case for better integration of care. Cureus. 2025;17:e83486.
74. Potter C, Feeney J, Fowler E, et al. Post-traumatic stress disorder and memory function in older adults exposed to civilian conflict: findings from the Northern Ireland Cohort for the Longitudinal Study of Ageing (NICOLA). Soc Sci Med. 2026;389:118840.
75. Rzeszutek M, Dragan M, Lis-Turlejska M, et al. Exposure to self-reported traumatic events and probable PTSD in a national sample of Poles: why does Poland's PTSD prevalence differ from other national estimates? PLoS One. 2023;18:e0287854.

76. Rzeszutek M, Dragan M, Lis-Turlejska M, et al. Adverse childhood experiences and ICD-11 complex posttraumatic stress disorder in Poland: a population-based study. Eur J Psychotraumatol; 15. Epub ahead of print 31 December 2024. https://doi.org/10.1080/20008066.2024.2420464.
77. Grieger TA, Fullerton CS, Ursano RJ. Posttraumatic stress disorder, alcohol use, and perceived safety after the terrorist attack on the Pentagon. 2003;54:1380–2.
78. Pulcino T, Galea S, Ahern J, et al. Posttraumatic stress in women after the September 11 terrorist attacks in New York City. J Women's Health. 2003;12:809–20.
79. Galea S, Ahern J, Resnick H, et al. Psychological sequelae of the September 11 terrorist attacks in New York City. N Engl J Med. 2002;346:982–7.
80. Fischer IC, Pietrzak RH, Maercker A, et al. Post-traumatic stress disorder: rethinking diagnosis. Lancet Psychiatry. 2023;10:741–2.
81. D'Andrea W, Chiu PH, Casas BR, et al. Linguistic predictors of post-traumatic stress disorder symptoms following 11 September 2001. Appl Cogn Psychol. 2012;26:316–23.
82. DiGrande L, Neria Y, Brackbill RM, et al. Long-term posttraumatic stress symptoms among 3,271 civilian survivors of the September 11, 2001, terrorist attacks on the World Trade Center. Am J Epidemiol. 2011;173:271–81.
83. Gargano LM, Nguyen A, DiGrande L, et al. Mental health status of World Trade Center tower survivors compared to other survivors a decade after the September 11, 2001 terrorist attacks. Am J Ind Med. 2016;59:742–51.
84. Ghafoori B, Neria Y, Gameroff MJ, et al. Screening for generalized anxiety disorder symptoms in the wake of terrorist attacks: a study in primary care. J Trauma Stress. 2009;22:218–26.
85. Xue J, Raitt J, Roaten K, et al. A study of suicidal thoughts and behaviour in a sample of adults affected by the 9/11 attacks on New York City's World Trade Center. Int Rev Psychiatry. 2022;34:89–96.
86. Sanz J, Hernández-Martínez T, Castillo-Burgos P, et al. Prevalence of increased alcohol use and alcohol use disorders in adult victims of terrorist attacks: a systematic and meta-analytic review. Am J Drug Alcohol Abuse. 2023;49:705–22.
87. Garrey SK, Welch AE, Jacobson MH, et al. The intentional self-medication of 9/11-related PTSD symptoms with alcohol: 15 years after the disaster. Int J Environ Res Public Health. 2020;17:5327.
88. Hirst A, Miller-Archie SA, Welch AE, et al. Post-9/11 drug- and alcohol-related hospitalizations among World Trade Center Health Registry enrollees, 2003–2010. Drug Alcohol Depend. 2018;187:55–60.
89. North CS, Adinoff B, Pollio DE, et al. Alcohol use disorders and drinking among survivors of the 9/11 attacks on the World Trade Center in New York City. Compr Psychiatry. 2013;54:962–9.
90. Takemoto E, Giesinger I, Russell JS, et al. Association between post-traumatic stress disorder and alcohol-related hospitalizations among World Trade Center Health Registry enrollees. Drug Alcohol Depend. 2021;221:108656.
91. Takemoto E, Brackbill R, Martins S, et al. Post-traumatic stress disorder and risk of prescription opioid use, over-use, and misuse among World Trade Center Health Registry enrollees, 2015–2016. Drug Alcohol Depend. 2020;210:107959.
92. Garrey SK, Locke S, Pollari C, et al. Post-traumatic stress disorder and risk of first-time and repeated opioid-related hospitalizations among World Trade Center Health Registry enrollees. Psychiatry Res. 2023;328:115462.
93. Liu R, Calvert GM, Anderson KR, et al. Opioid prescriptions among the World Trade Center Health Program population. BMC Health Serv Res. 2023;23:1323.
94. Dhanya AS, Yung J, Cone JE, et al. Association of rheumatoid arthritis with opioid pain medication overuse among persons exposed to the 9/11 World Trade Center disaster. Int J Environ Res Public Health. 2023;20:4166.
95. Keefe PR. Empire of pain. Doubleday; 2021.

96. North CS, Pfefferbaum B. Tobacco and illicit drug use and drug use disorders among employees of businesses affected by the 9/11 attacks on the World Trade Center in New York City. J Dual Diagn. 2023;19:180–8.
97. North CS, Nixon SJ, Shariat S, et al. Psychiatric disorders among survivors of the Oklahoma City bombing. JAMA. 1999;282:755.
98. North CS, McDonald K, Pollio DE. A longitudinal follow-up study of Oklahoma City bombing survivors in the first quarter century after the disaster. Ann Clin Psychiatry. 2023;35:93–100.
99. Tucker P, Pfefferbaum B, Watson K, et al. Problems and needs persist for Oklahoma City bombing survivors many years later. Behav Sci. 2021;11:19.
100. Koenen KC, Ratanatharathorn A, Ng L, et al. Posttraumatic stress disorder in the World Mental Health Surveys. Psychol Med. 2017;47:2260–74.
101. Kessler RC, Aguilar-Gaxiola S, Alonso J, et al. Trauma and PTSD in the WHO world mental health surveys. Eur J Psychotraumatol; 8. Epub ahead of print 27 October 2017. https://doi.org/10.1080/20008198.2017.1353383.
102. Solberg Ø, Blix I, Heir T. The aftermath of terrorism: posttraumatic stress and functional impairment after the 2011 Oslo bombing. Front Psychol; 6. Epub ahead of print 7 August 2015. https://doi.org/10.3389/fpsyg.2015.01156.
103. Dyb G, Jensen TK, Nygaard E, et al. Post-traumatic stress reactions in survivors of the 2011 massacre on Utøya Island, Norway. Br J Psychiatry. 2014;204:361–7.
104. Aakvaag HF, Thoresen S, Wentzel-Larsen T, et al. Shame and guilt in the aftermath of terror: the Utøya Island study. J Trauma Stress. 2014;27:618–21.
105. Undset A, Jensen T, Birkeland MS, et al. Maladaptive appraisals and posttraumatic stress reactions in young terror survivors across 8 years: a random intercepts cross-lagged analysis. Eur J Psychotraumatol; 16. Epub ahead of print 31 December 2025. https://doi.org/10.1080/20008066.2025.2459462.
106. Glad KA, Porcheret K, Dyb G. Prevalence and potency of trauma reminders 8.5 years after a terrorist attack. Eur J Psychotraumatol; 14. Epub ahead of print 23 November 2023. https://doi.org/10.1080/20008066.2023.2251774.
107. Glad KA, Jensen TK, Hafstad GS, et al. Posttraumatic stress disorder and exposure to trauma reminders after a terrorist attack. J Trauma Dissoc. 2016;17:435–47.
108. Glad KA, Hafstad GS, Jensen TK, et al. A longitudinal study of psychological distress and exposure to trauma reminders after terrorism. Psychol Trauma. 2017;9:145–52.
109. Porcheret K, Dyb G, Wentzel-Larsen T, et al. Predictors of early adulthood insomnia following exposure to a single mass violence attack during adolescence: 7–13 year follow-up from the Utøya and HUNT studies. Eur J Psychotraumatol; 15. Epub ahead of print 31 December 2024. https://doi.org/10.1080/20008066.2024.2312750.
110. Porcheret K, Stensland SØ, Wentzel-Larsen T, et al. Insomnia in survivors 8.5 years after the Utøya Island terrorist attack: transition from late adolescence to early adulthood – the Utøya study. Eur J Psychotraumatol. 2022;13:2020472.
111. Nordström E-EL, Kaltiala R, Kristensen P, et al. Somatic symptoms and insomnia among bereaved parents and siblings eight years after the Utøya terror attack. Eur J Psychotraumatol; 15. Epub ahead of print 31 December 2024. https://doi.org/10.1080/20008066.2023.2300585
.
112. Gómez de La Cuesta G, Schweizer S, Diehle J, et al. The relationship between maladaptive appraisals and posttraumatic stress disorder: a meta-analysis. Eur J Psychotraumatol; 10. Epub ahead of print 31 December 2019. https://doi.org/10.1080/20008198.2019.1620084.
113. Filkuková P, Hafstad GS, Jensen TK. Who can I trust? Extended fear during and after the Utøya terrorist attack. Psychol Trauma. 2016;8:512–9.
114. Nilsen LG, Thoresen S, Wentzel-Larsen T, et al. Trust after terror: institutional trust among young terror survivors and their parents after the 22nd of July terrorist attack on Utøya Island, Norway. Front Psychol; 10. Epub ahead of print 13 December 2019. https://doi.org/10.3389/fpsyg.2019.02819.

115. Stensland SØ, Zwart J-A, Wentzel-Larsen T, et al. The headache of terror. Neurology; 90. Epub ahead of print 9 January 2018. https://doi.org/10.1212/WNL.0000000000004805.
116. Stubberud A, Buse DC, Kristoffersen ES, et al. Is there a causal relationship between stress and migraine? Current evidence and implications for management. J Headache Pain. 2021;22:155.
117. Stensland SØ, Thoresen S, Jensen T, et al. Early pain and other somatic symptoms predict posttraumatic stress reactions in survivors of terrorist attacks: the longitudinal Utøya Cohort study. J Trauma Stress. 2020;33:1060–70.
118. Holt T, Jensen T, Dyb G, et al. Emotional reactions in parents of the youth who experienced the Utøya shooting on 22 July 2011; results from a cohort study. BMJ Open. 2017;7:e015345.
119. Thoresen S, Jensen TK, Wentzel-Larsen T, et al. Parents of terror victims. A longitudinal study of parental mental health following the 2011 terrorist attack on Utøya Island. J Anxiety Disord. 2016;38:47–54.
120. Glad KA, Czajkowski NO, Dyb G, et al. Does event centrality mediate the effect of peritraumatic reactions on post-traumatic growth in survivors of a terrorist attack? Eur J Psychotraumatol. 2020;11:1766276.
121. Kristensen P, Dyregrov K, Dyregrov A. Can visiting the site of death be beneficial for bereaved families after terror? A qualitative study of parents' and siblings' experiences of visiting Utøya Island after the 2011 Norway terror attack. Eur J Psychotraumatol; 8 Epub ahead of print 29 December 2017. https://doi.org/10.1080/20008198.2018.1463795.
122. Bell C, Sulaiman-Hill R, Tanveer S, et al. Factors associated with mental health outcomes in a Muslim community following the Christchurch terrorist attack. BJPsych Open. 2024;10:e209.
123. Byrne KG, Yogeeswaran K, Dorahy MJ, et al. Psychological impact of far-right terrorism against Muslim minorities on national distress, community, and wellbeing. Sci Rep. 2022;12:1620.
124. Dean S, Eggleston K, Ali F, et al. 'I can feel sad about it and I can worry, but inside I know everything happens for a reason': personal experiences in the aftermath of the March 15 Christchurch mosque attacks. BJPsych Open. 2024;10:e176.
125. Beaglehole B, Boden JM, Porter R, et al. Post-traumatic growth and religious coping in Muslims exposed to the March 15 terror attacks in New Zealand: a cross-sectional study. Austral N Zeal J Psychiatry; Epub ahead of print 16 September 2025. https://doi.org/10.1177/00048674251374461.
126. Duffy M, McDermott M, Percy A, et al. The effects of the Omagh bomb on adolescent mental health: a school-based study. BMC Psychiatry. 2015;15:18.
127. Duffy M, Bolton D, Gillespie K, et al. A community study of the psychological effects of the Omagh car bomb on adults. PLoS One. 2013;8:e76618.
128. Zhang G, North CS, Narayanan P, et al. The course of postdisaster psychiatric disorders in directly exposed civilians after the US Embassy bombing in Nairobi, Kenya: a follow-up study. Soc Psychiatry Psychiatr Epidemiol. 2013;48:195–203.
129. North CS, Dvorkina T, Thielman S, et al. A study of selected ethnic affiliations in the development of post-traumatic stress disorder and other psychopathology after a terrorist bombing in Nairobi, Kenya. Disaster Med Public Health Prep. 2018;12:360–5.
130. Raitt JM, Thielman SB, Pfefferbaum B, et al. Psychosocial effects on US Government personnel of exposure to the 1998 terrorist attack on the US Embassy in Nairobi. Psychiatry. 2021;84:165–81.
131. Gobin M, Rubin GJ, Albert I, et al. Outcomes of mental health screening for United Kingdom nationals affected by the 2015–2016 terrorist attacks in Tunisia, Paris, and Brussels. J Trauma Stress. 2018;31:471–9.
132. Cyhlarova E, Knapp M, Mays N. Responding to the mental health consequences of the 2015–2016 terrorist attacks in Tunisia, Paris and Brussels: implementation and treatment experiences in the United Kingdom. J Health Serv Res Policy. 2020;25:172–80.
133. Handley RV, Salkovskis PM, Ehlers A. Treating clinically significant avoidance of public transport following the London bombings? Behav Cogn Psychother. 2009;37:87–93.

134. Handley RV, Salkovskis PM, Scragg P, et al. Clinically significant avoidance of public transport following the London bombings: travel phobia or subthreshold posttraumatic stress disorder? J Anxiety Disord. 2009;23:1170–6.
135. Fullerton CS, Herberman Mash HB, Benevides KN, et al. Distress of routine activities and perceived safety associated with post-traumatic stress, depression, and alcohol use: 2002 Washington, DC, sniper attacks. Disaster Med Public Health Prep. 2015;9:509–15.
136. Conejo-Galindo J, Medina Ó, Fraguas D, et al. Psychopathological sequelae of the 11 March terrorist attacks in Madrid. Eur Arch Psychiatry Clin Neurosci. 2007;258:28–34.
137. Gabriel R, Ferrando L, Cortón ES, et al. Psychopathological consequences after a terrorist attack: an epidemiological study among victims, the general population, and police officers. Eur Psychiatry. 2007;22:339–46.
138. Fausor R, Sanz J, Navarro-McCarthy A, et al. Long-term posttraumatic growth in victims of terrorism in Spain. Front Psychol. 2022;13:847099.
139. Zara A. Grief intensity, coping and psychological health among family members and friends following a terrorist attack. Death Stud. 2020;44:366–74.
140. Eşsizoğlu A, Altınöz AE, Sonkurt HO, et al. The risk factors of possible PTSD in individuals exposed to a suicide attack in Turkey. Psychiatry Res. 2017;253:274–80.
141. Sugiyama A, Matsuoka T, Sakamune K, et al. The Tokyo subway sarin attack has long-term effects on survivors: a 10-year study started 5 years after the terrorist incident. PLoS One. 2020;15:e0234967.
142. Kawana N, Ishimatsu S, Kanda K. Psycho-physiological effects of the terrorist sarin attack on the Tokyo subway system. Mil Med. 2001;166:23–6.
143. Moscardino U, Scrimin S, Capello F, et al. Psychological adjustment of adolescents 18 months after the terrorist attack in Beslan, Russia. J Clin Psychiatry. 2008;69:854–9.
144. Scrimin S, Moscardino U, Capello F, et al. Trauma reminders and PTSD symptoms in children three years after a terrorist attack in Beslan. Soc Sci Med. 2011;72:694–700.
145. Moscardino U, Scrimin S, Capello F, et al. Are Beslan's children learning to cope? J Clin Psychiatry. 2011;72:1277–83.
146. Moscardino U, Scrimin S, Capello F, et al. Social support, sense of community, collectivistic values, and depressive symptoms in adolescent survivors of the 2004 Beslan terrorist attack. Soc Sci Med. 2010;70:27–34.
147. Scrimin S, Axia G, Capello F, et al. Posttraumatic reactions among injured children and their caregivers 3 months after the terrorist attack in Beslan. Psychiatry Res. 2006;141:333–6.
148. Balasinorwala VP, Shah N. Acute stress disorder in victims after terror attacks in Mumbai, India. Br J Psychiatry. 2009;195:462.
149. Balasinorwala VP, Shah N. Acute stress disorder in hospitalised victims of 26/11-terror attack on Mumbai, India. J Indian Med Assoc. 2010;108(757):759–60.
150. Banerjee AV, Esther D. Poor economics: the surprising truth about life on less than $1 a day. Penguin Books; 2012.
151. Lavi T, Solomon Z. Palestinian youth of the Intifada: PTSD and future orientation. J Am Acad Child Adolesc Psychiatry. 2005;44:1176–83.
152. Solomon Z, Lavi T. Israeli youth in the second Intifada: PTSD and future orientation. J Am Acad Child Adolesc Psychiatry. 2005;44:1167–75.
153. Di Maio M, Leone SV. Conflict exposure and health: evidence from the Gaza Strip. Health Econ. 2021;30:2287–95.
154. Hamama-Raz Y, Solomon Z, Cohen A, et al. PTSD symptoms, forgiveness, and revenge among Israeli Palestinian and Jewish adolescents. J Trauma Stress. 2008;21:521–9.
155. Ayer L, Venkatesh B, Stewart R, et al. Psychological aspects of the Israeli–Palestinian conflict: a systematic review. Trauma Violence Abuse. 2017;18:322–38.
156. Rosenberg A, Heimberg RG, Solomon Z, et al. Investigation of exposure–symptom relationships in a context of recurrent violence. J Anxiety Disord. 2008;22:416–28.
157. Eran-Jona M, Tiargan-Orr R, Levine SZ, et al. Habituation of fear—Israeli-Jewish population during protracted belligerence. Int J Environ Res Public Health. 2022;19:16067.

158. Bleich A, Gelkopf M, Melamed Y, et al. Mental health and resiliency following 44 months of terrorism: a survey of an Israeli national representative sample. BMC Med. 2006;4:21.
159. Bleich A. Exposure to terrorism, stress-related mental health symptoms, and coping behaviors among a nationally representative sample in Israel. JAMA. 2003;290:612.
160. Gidron Y, Kaplan Y, Velt A, et al. Prevalence and moderators of terror-related post-traumatic stress disorder symptoms in Israeli citizens. Isr Med Assoc J. 2004;6:387–91.
161. Pat-Horenczyk R, Peled O, Miron T, et al. Risk-taking behaviors among Israeli adolescents exposed to recurrent terrorism: provoking danger under continuous threat? Am J Psychiatry. 2007;164:66–72.
162. Pat-Horenczyk R, Abramovitz R, Peled O, et al. Adolescent exposure to recurrent terrorism in Israel: posttraumatic distress and functional impairment. Am J Orthopsychiatry. 2007;77:76–85.
163. Kalanthroff E, Berebbi S, David M, et al. Acute trauma and obsessive compulsive disorder: evidence from October 7th. Psychother Psychosom. 2023;2025:1–12.
164. Groweiss Y, Blank C, Hamdan S, et al. The mental health impact of the October 7th terror attack on Jews and Arabs in Israel: a nationwide prospective study. Psychiatry Res. 2024;337:115973.
165. Mayer Y, Shiffman N, Bergmann E, et al. Mental health outcomes of Arab and Jewish populations in Israel a month after the mass trauma events of October 7, 2023: a cross-sectional survey of a representative sample. Psychiatry Res. 2024;339:116042.
166. Levi-Belz Y, Amsalem D, Groweiss Y, et al. The role of PTSD-depression comorbidity in long-term mental health sequalae of the October 7th terror attack in Israel: a nationwide prospective study. J Affect Disord. 2025;381:410–7.
167. Chemtob CM, Pat-Horenczyk R, Madan A, et al. Israeli adolescents with ongoing exposure to terrorism: suicidal ideation, posttraumatic stress disorder, and functional impairment. J Trauma Stress. 2011;24:756–9.
168. Feingold D, Neria Y, Bitan DT. PTSD, distress and substance use in the aftermath of October 7th, 2023, terror attacks in Southern Israel. J Psychiatr Res. 2024;174:153–8.
169. Eliashar R, Zilberstein T, Shmulewitz D, et al. Reported increase in substance use following mass terrorism and the role of psychosocial factors. JAMA Netw Open. 2024;7:e2423993.
170. Massey Z, Chartier KG, Stebbins MB, et al. Explaining the frequency of alcohol consumption in a conflict zone: Jews and Palestinians in Israel. Addict Behav. 2015;46:31–8.
171. Cohen M, Eid J. The effect of constant threat of terror on Israeli Jewish and Arab adolescents. Anxiety Stress Coping. 2007;20:47–60.
172. Gelkopf M, Solomon Z, Berger R, et al. The mental health impact of terrorism in Israel: a repeat cross-sectional study of Arabs and Jews. Acta Psychiatr Scand. 2008;117:369–80.
173. Shechory Bitton M, Silawi Y. Do Jews and Arabs differ in their fear of terrorism and crime? J Interpers Violence. 2019;34:4041–60.
174. Kaplan G, Glasser S, Murad H, et al. Depression among Arabs and Jews in Israel: a population-based study. Soc Psychiatry Psychiatr Epidemiol. 2010;45:931–9.
175. Braun-Lewensohn O, Sagy S. Coping resources as explanatory factors of stress reactions during missile attacks: comparing Jewish and Arab adolescents in Israel. Community Ment Health J. 2011;47:300–10.
176. Braun-Lewensohn O, Sagy S, Roth G. Coping strategies among adolescents: Israeli Jews and Arabs facing missile attacks. Anxiety Stress Coping. 2010;23:35–51.
177. Abu-Kaf S, Braun-Lewensohn O. Coping resources and stress reactions among Bedouin Arab adolescents during three military operations. Psychiatry Res. 2019;273:559–66.
178. Eshel Y, Kimhi S, Marciano H, et al. Ethnic origin of Israeli Jews and psychological responses to the extreme stress of the ongoing war with Hamas in Gaza. Front Psychol; 15. Epub ahead of print 23 October 2024. https://doi.org/10.3389/fpsyg.2024.1403132.
179. Van Overmeire R, Vesentini L, Van Keer R-L, et al. Working experiences of airport employees after a terrorist attack in Belgium: a qualitative study. Int J Disaster Risk Reduct. 2021;64:102515.

180. Schouten R, Callahan MV, Bryant S. Community response to disaster: the role of the workplace. Harv Rev Psychiatry. 2004;12:229–37.
181. North CS, Pfefferbaum B, Hong BA, et al. Workplace response of companies exposed to the 9/11 World Trade Center attack: a focus-group study. Disasters. 2013;37:101–18.
182. Miu AS, Davis AJ, Raitt JM, et al. Employee job satisfaction and performance in association with workplace responses to the 9/11 attacks on New York City's World Trade Center. J Occup Environ Med. 2022;64:115–22.
183. North CS, Pfefferbaum B, Hong BA, et al. The business of healing: focus group discussions of readjustment to the post-9/11 work environment among employees of affected agencies. J Occup Environ Med. 2010;52:713–8.
184. Birkeland MS, Nielsen MB, Knardahl S, et al. Time-lagged relationships between leadership behaviors and psychological distress after a workplace terrorist attack. Int Arch Occup Environ Health. 2016;89:689–97.
185. Nissen A, Birkeland Nielsen M, Solberg Ø, et al. Perception of threat and safety at work among employees in the Norwegian ministries after the 2011 Oslo bombing. Anxiety Stress Coping. 2015;28:650–62.
186. North CS, Barney CJ, Pollio DE. A focus group study of the impact of trauma exposure in the 9/11 terrorist attacks. Soc Psychiatry Psychiatr Epidemiol. 2015;50:569–78.
187. Waldrep D, Waits W. Returning to the Pentagon: the use of mass desensitization following the September 11, 2001 attack. Mil Med. 2002;167:58–9.
188. Hoge CW, Orman DT, Robichaux RJ, et al. Operation Solace: overview of the mental health intervention following the September 11, 2001 Pentagon attack. Mil Med. 2002;167:44–7.
189. Milliken CS, Leavitt WT, Murdock P, et al. Principles guiding implementation of the Operation Solace plan: 'Pieces of PIES,' therapy by walking around, and care management. Mil Med. 2002;167:48–57.
190. Tarpley AA. A perspective on the Air Force's mental health response to the Pentagon. Mil Med. 2002;167:26–30.
191. Van Overmeire R, Muysewinkel E, Van Keer R-L, et al. Victims of the terrorist attacks in Belgium and professional mental health aid barriers: a qualitative study Front Psychiatry; 12. Epub ahead of print 2 July 2021. https://doi.org/10.3389/fpsyt.2021.638272.
192. Jordan NN, Hoge CW, Tobler SK, et al. Mental health impact of 9/11 Pentagon attack. Am J Prev Med. 2004;26:284–93.
193. Grieger TA, Waldrep DA, Lovasz MM, et al. Follow-up of Pentagon employees two years after the terrorist attack of September 11, 2001. 2005;56:1374–8.
194. North CS, Pollio DE, Smith RP, et al. Trauma exposure and posttraumatic stress disorder among employees of New York City companies affected by the September 11, 2001 attacks on the World Trade Center. Disaster Med Public Health Prep. 2011;5:S205–13.
195. Reynolds ME, Raitt JM, Üstyol A, et al. Personality and psychiatric disorders among employees of New York City workplaces affected by the 9/11 attacks on the World Trade Center. Psychiatry. 2022;85:38–55.
196. Birkeland MS, Heir T. Making connections: exploring the centrality of posttraumatic stress symptoms and covariates after a terrorist attack. Eur J Psychotraumatol; 8. Epub ahead of print 30 November 2017. https://doi.org/10.1080/20008198.2017.1333387.
197. Solberg Ø, Birkeland MS, Blix I, et al. Towards an exposure-dependent model of post-traumatic stress: longitudinal course of post-traumatic stress symptomatology and functional impairment after the 2011 Oslo bombing. Psychol Med. 2016;46:3241–54.
198. Hansen MB, Berthelsen M, Nissen A, et al. Sick leave before and after a work-place targeted terror attack. Int Arch Occup Environ Health. 2019;92:327–35.
199. Berthelsen M, Hansen MB, Nissen A, et al. Effects of exposure to workplace terrorism on subsequent doctor certified sickness absence, and the modifying role of psychological and social work factors: a combined survey and register study. BMC Public Health. 2020;20:367.
200. Boscarino JA, Adams RE, Figley CR. Worker productivity and outpatient service use after the September 11th attacks: results from the New York City Terrorism Outcome Study. Am J Ind Med. 2006;49:670–82.

201. Dale MTG, Nissen A, Berthelsen M, et al. Post-traumatic stress reactions and doctor-certified sick leave after a workplace terrorist attack: Norwegian cohort study. BMJ Open. 2020;10:e032693.
202. Nissen A, Berthelsen M, Dale MTG, et al. Is perceived safety and threat after workplace terrorism linked to employee sick-leave? A registry-based longitudinal study of governmental employees in Norway. Eur J Psychotraumatol; 11. Epub ahead of print 31 December 2020. https://doi.org/10.1080/20008198.2020.1785249.
203. Dale MTG, Nissen A, Berthelsen M, et al. Psychosocial work factors and sick leave risk after a terrorist bomb attack: a survey and registry-based longitudinal study of governmental employees in Norway. BMJ Open. 2021;11:e052628.
204. Birkeland MS, Nielsen MB, Hansen MB, et al. Like a bridge over troubled water? A longitudinal study of general social support, colleague support, and leader support as recovery factors after a traumatic event. Eur J Psychotraumatol; 8. Epub ahead of print 1 January 2017. https://doi.org/10.1080/20008198.2017.1302692.
205. Berthelsen M, Hansen MB, Nissen A, et al. The impact of a workplace terrorist attack on the psychosocial work environment: a longitudinal study from pre- to post-disaster. Front Public Health; 9. Epub ahead of print 4 November 2021. https://doi.org/10.3389/fpubh.2021.708260.
206. Birkeland MS, Nielsen MB, Knardahl S, et al. Associations between work environment and psychological distress after a workplace terror attack: the importance of role expectations, predictability and leader support. PLoS One. 2015;10:e0119492.
207. Hem C, Nielsen MB, Hansen MB, et al. Effort-reward imbalance and post-traumatic stress after a workplace terror attack. Disaster Med Public Health Prep. 2016;10:219–24.
208. Heir T, Stokke EH, Tvenge KP. The role of workplace on work participation and sick leave after a terrorist attack: a qualitative study. Int J Environ Res Public Health. 2021;18:1920.
209. Hansen MB, Nissen A, Heir T. Proximity to terror and post-traumatic stress: a follow-up survey of governmental employees after the 2011 Oslo bombing attack. BMJ Open. 2013;3:e002692.
210. Nissen A, Hansen MB, Nielsen MB, et al. Employee safety perception following workplace terrorism: a longitudinal study. Eur J Psychotraumatol; 10. Epub ahead of print 31 December 2019. https://doi.org/10.1080/20008198.2018.1478584.

# Chapter 3
# Running Towards the Danger: Rescue Workers and Their Mental Health After Terrorist Attacks

## 3.1 Introduction

The previous chapter (Chap. 2) concerned people directly exposed to terrorist attacks. It is important to differentiate this group from those who are also directly exposed to terrorist attacks in their professional capacity, because despite sharing exposure, the consequences and context is completely different for this group. In this chapter, this group who in their professional capacity react to a disaster such as a terrorist attack, will be called "rescue workers" throughout, despite synonyms like first responders, emergency responders, and other terms [1].

Defining a broad group such as rescue workers is best done through examples: firefighters, ambulance personnel, police officers, etc. These are people who respond to a mass traumatic event, in order to help survivors, and/or to eliminate the remaining threats.

The reason for making a separate chapter on rescue workers is due to several reasons. First, an old motto of rescue workers is "When people run away from danger, we run towards it," which highlights the difference between the survivors discussed in Chap. 2 and rescue worker: rescue workers have specific roles during a crisis; in fact, it is their job to act in a crisis. That is a completely different psychological mindset compared to those of people going to work or on vacation, people who have jobs and lives unrelated to crises, but who are put into a disaster.

Second, rescue workers, at least professional ones, often have their own support network. Rescue workers go into a disaster together; they go out of it together [2]. In the case of firefighters, ambulance personnel, military personnel, and other rescue worker groups, rescue workers see each other on a constant basis. They have a group bond, which can be a protective or negative thing, but it certainly differentiates them from individual civilian survivors.


R. Van Overmeire, *Terrorism, Mental Health and Aftercare*,
https://doi.org/10.1007/978-3-032-31560-1_3

## 3.2 Note on the Findings

As with Chap. 2, a general problem of making a summary of findings is the fragmentation of findings. One database is cut into numerous articles, which is sometimes done not out of the idea of focusing on one aspect of a population, but out of the idea of having more publications. This fragmentation sometimes hampers coming to proper findings, and it is sometimes a puzzle to create a grander picture and provide clear, overall conclusions.

Also important to note is that post-traumatic stress disorder (PTSD) is here too the most important outcome. As discussed broadly in Chap. 1, such outcomes are sometimes measured in a puzzling way. Furthermore, sometimes samples of rescue workers take together those who are not directly exposed [3]. Other studies might actually simply never measure the exposure to a disaster, and simply assume direct exposure. Related to PTSD as outcome is the importance that PTSD is also related to changing memories. For example, one longitudinal study showed that after 9/11 showed that throughout time, 51% of respondents had changed their perception whether the smells during and after the attack had been traumatic for them [4]. In other words, even in longitudinal studies, memories of the events will change, and perhaps affect outcomes.

Due to aspects that are inherent to public health research, such as differences in samples, measurement tools, and timing, rates for the same population might differ quite a lot. Furthermore, as with all studies in this book, self-reported measures are the standard, and these have the tendency to overestimate, but also most samples are voluntary samples, which might mean that people join a sample because they have most mental health issues [1]. Additionally, such self-reported surveys in convenience samples give a higher prevalence of mental health problems [5].

Finally, as a note on the terrorist attacks in this chapter, the reader should also be aware that while many terrorist attacks are mentioned, they are often not described in terms of the actual attack. For reference, the reader can find a list of terrorist attacks in the Appendix that describes, in short, the nature of the attack.

## 3.3 Mental Health Issues Among Rescue Workers

In general, rescue workers have fewer mental health issues than the general population. Overall, for PTSD, the prevalence among rescue workers is worldwide estimated at around 10% [6, 7], while for rescue workers after terrorist attacks the range is much bigger. One systematic review estimated PTSD being between 1.3% and 16.5% [1]. While lower than the general population (which is estimated more around 30–40% for PTSD [8, 9]), the difference is, and this is true especially for rescue workers who were exposed to terrorist attacks, that the PTSD tends to be more often chronic than in the general population [1]. This means that while the

PTSD rates are higher survivors, they also decrease more compared to rescue workers with PTSD.

It is difficult to provide an estimate of the prevalence of PTSD or mental health problems in rescue workers in relation to terrorist attacks, as there are many different factors at place, such as the type of terrorist attack, and of course cultural and social factors [6]. Thus, there are quite large differences depending on the attacks. For example, rescue workers after the Madrid Bombing or the London attacks had very low PTSD and depression rates (1–4%) [10, 11], while in the USA and France these were at times more than three times as high (8–12%) [1, 12, 13].

It is made even more difficult due to the issue of the late onset of PTSD, and the fluctuating nature of PTSD, where symptoms can be worse or fade depending on the time [14]. For example, in the case of 9/11, the rates of PTSD were higher 4–5 years after the attacks compared to how they were 2–3 years after the attacks [1]. This ensures that any measure of mental health problems is nuanced. Hence, percentages should always be viewed with nuance.

There are numerous factors that are correlated with mental health issues among rescue workers, including pre-disaster factors, during disaster factors, and post-disaster factors [15].

### 3.3.1 Pre-terrorism Factors

**Background Factors**

Certain factors, such as age and gender, also play a role in the risk of developing mental health issues among rescue workers. Studies after 9/11, for example, found that women rescue workers had a higher chance of developing PTSD, as well as those that are older, and those of Hispanic descent [16–18]. Gender wise, it seems that women are more at risk than men to develop mental health issues [16]. For example, among police officers, while the average PTSD percentage was roughly 8%, this was 13% for female police officers [16]. There is also seemingly a difference in how symptoms exhibit themselves. Studies in Germany show that male rescue workers became more paranoid than female rescue workers [19–21].

**Preparedness and Operation Factors:**

A major difference with civilians exposed to terrorism is the factor of operational factors: occupation, role, training, teamwork, communication, etc [22]. In fact, while few studies have looked into operational factors, these factors can be better predictors of mental health than background factors such as gender or age [11]. One study after the 2015 Paris attacks, for example, showed that a lack of training, and the fear related to interventions in unsecured crime scenes where terrorists might still be present, were indicative of PTSD [23]. Other studies, after the Brussels attacks or the Manchester attacks, showed that operational factors such as communication can also be related to distress and fear [2, 24, 25].

The role of experience and, especially, training, is important is negating negative effects of exposure to terrorist attacks. For example, Norwegian rescue workers had very low PTSD rates (1.3% 8–11 months after, dropping to 0.3%) [26, 27], but almost all had previous experience, and most involved knew their roles [27, 28]. A nuance, which again shows to the difficulty of interpretation, is that a study on rescue workers in Norway in non-terrorist times showed actually higher PTSD and depression rates than after the terrorist attacks [29].

However, the role of preparation and the knowing of roles is also reflected in other studies [2]. For example, the relatively low rate of mental problems among rescue workers after the 2005 bombings in England might be explained by the staff knowing the post-disaster plans for mental health aid [11]. While 31% of the general population had severe distress after the attacks, this was only 13% among the rescue workers, and only 4% had probably PTSD [11, 30].

### *3.3.2 During Terrorism*

**Exposure**

As might be obvious, exposure to the terrorist attack plays a critical role in predicting mental health issues among rescue workers [31, 32]. For example, one study showed that healthcare emergency staff that were involved in the rescue operation during the Paris attacks had double as much risk to develop PTSD compared to colleagues who had not been involved in the rescue operation [33]. Similarly, after the Strasbourg attack in 2018, police officers exposed to the violence had more PTSD than those not exposed. However, interestingly, the relation was absent for depression, where both exposed and non-exposed groups had equal chance of developing it, indicating the role of exposure for PTSD [34].

**Related Health Issues**

Another factor are diseases due to the exposure, which is most relevant in the context of 9/11. For example, the high incidence of PTSD among rescue workers after 9/11 might also be due to factors such as the asbestos and other materials that were set loose when the towers crashed, which is associated with cancer (though, it should be noted, this incidence is lower than expected) [35–38]. Similarly, rescue workers involved with the 9/11 rescue operations have more asthma than the general population, possibly due to the dust clouds [39] or hearing problems [40]. Such problems are correlated with PTSD [31, 41, 42]. This relation between dust, asbestos, and mental health is not always relevant in other rescue workers—for example, rescue workers after a terrorist shooting will face other issues.

**Situational Factors**

Furthermore, while rescue workers have lower risk for mental health issues than the general population [43], there are factors that make them equally vulnerable, such as losing colleagues during the action, or, in the case of 9/11, being stuck in the dust cloud after the towers collapsed… [13, 44]. In the case of other disasters, such as

Oklahoma City Bombing and the Brussels attacks, during the rescue operation, there was a constant threat of someone who might attack [2, 22].

The subjective threat that rescue workers feel during the action is an important indicator of future mental health problems [45]. For example, one study on Pakistani emergency personnel after a terrorist attack showed that 15% had PTSD, but that this was not related to the size of the attack, but more to the sense of threat the rescue workers felt [46]. A study after 9/11 showed that this sense of safety, or lack of it, was indicative of PTSD even weeks after 9/11 for disaster workers at the site of the Twin Towers [45].

The majority of the rescue workers in Norway saw dead or injured people, but few (5.7%) saw it as extremely stressful [26]. In fact, the rescue workers most at risk were those who were unaffiliated volunteers [27].

Another factor is the feeling of guilt during the action. For example, some rescue workers might feel guilty due to not being able to come into action during that day, or feel guilty for not having performed well [2, 22]. In addition, rescue workers often have to try and save as many people as they can. However, in an emergency disaster setting, resources are limited. As such, time and energy should only be given to those who have the highest chance of surviving, instead of those that seem to take too much time and resources [2, 22]. This economic efficiency decision that has to be made on the spot can lead to severe guilt and can be associated with mental health issues later on [47].

### 3.3.3 *Post-terrorism*

**Additional Exposure to Disasters**

It could be argued that the work of rescue workers is essentially exposure to disasters. As such, the further exposure to disasters after a terrorist attack can contribute to mental health issues. For example, around 6% of retired firefighters, roughly 3 years after 9/11, had PTSD [48], while in the same time period, the amount of still active firefighters had roughly 15% [49]. Other studies found that especially among non-professional rescue workers (e.g. volunteers) this was especially the case [17]. This also works in the reverse: previous trauma, as well as previous mental health issues, can be predictive of PTSD [50]. For example, among health service staff after the 1998 Omagh bombing in Northern Ireland, previous trauma exposure was predictive of PTSD [51]. However, among utility workers with PTSD, half had, in addition to no psychiatric history, no previous trauma exposure, showcasing that this is certainly not a golden rule [52].

**Substance Abuse**

A common coping strategy after terrorism is the abuse of substances. For example, after the attacks in Norway, despite having low PTSD rates among rescue workers, those who did have PTSD were often also using medicinal drugs or drinking more alcohol [53]. Additionally, rescue workers active during the Oklahoma City

Bombing drank more alcohol to cope, though this might also already have been the case before the bombing itself [54, 55]. Such substance abuse is correlated with more mental health issues. While smoking in general is a common way of coping after terrorist attacks, one study among police officers after 9/11 showed that smoking could be linked with more PTSD [56]. Such substance abuse leads not just to mental health issues, but also to decreased social functioning, leading to job loss (which in turn leads to a decreased access to healthcare) and social and personal problems [56, 57].

**Low Social Support**
Perceiving little support from colleagues, friends, and family generally will lead to a higher risk of developing PTSD after exposure to terrorist attacks [1]. Social support is a complex issue, that will be discussed in a later chapter more in-depth. However, suffice to say, an attack affects the routines and can affect relationships. In the case of rescue workers, this can be that friends and family, or even the partners, also have to cope [58] with the event, or that there is a lack of understanding of the social support [59]. In addition, it might also be, of course, that some rescue workers had little social support even before the attack, which would mean that they would not have the necessary support after the attacks, yet this is important, considering that social support is one of the most important protective factors against the development of PTSD and other mental health issues [59].

Additionally, what plays more a role in rescue workers opposed to the general population is the stronger stigma for mental health. A rescue worker often feels they need to be "strong" and reflect traditional ideas on masculinity [11], yet mental health issues might lead to pushing social support away, and end in social isolation [1].

## 3.4 Differences Between Types of Rescue Workers

There are two main observations on the differences between rescue workers.

First, professional rescue workers are more resilient than non-professional rescue workers.

Second, professional firefighters will in general be more resilient than other professional rescue workers.

### *3.4.1 Professional Versus Non-professional*

Under non-professional rescue workers fall those people who are either (1) volunteer rescue worker, and thus mainly come into action when extra rescue workers are needed; (2) those who, due to the nature of their job, have to be at a scene of a disaster, but have no training in anything related to rescue workers; for example, utility workers or construction workers [52, 60–63].

Studies have shown that after 9/11, police officers were more resilient than non-traditional rescue workers, such as construction workers [62, 63]. Similarly, rescue workers intervening in the 1998 Nairobi ambassade bombing had much higher PTSD rates than those after the Oklahoma City Bombing, which might be due to the fact that they were mostly volunteers [64]. In fact, the Nairobi rescue workers had roughly the same rates as the citizens exposed to the bombing, indicating that they did not have the usual protective factors that rescue workers have due to their training and experience [64].

There are few studies overall that have used clinical interviews on rescue workers. A clinical interview is when someone is interviewed by a psychologist rather than completing a self-reported questionnaire; it is generally seen as more reliable, though doubts about this being a gold standard are expressed in Chap. 1. Two of these studies also show the stark difference between professional groups. One on firefighters after 9/11 showed that 6.5% had PTSD [48], while among utility workers this was initially 14.9% [65]. However, an important nuance here is that the 14.9% dropped to 5.8% 7 years after the attacks [65].

Similarly, after the attacks in Norway, few of the rescue workers experienced the seeing of dead bodies or injured people as stressful; the exception being the unaffiliated volunteers, who were distressed by the events and sights [26, 27]. Furthermore, while the professional rescue workers hardly used sick days, nor used alcohol, drugs, or medicine to cope after attacks, the volunteers did [53, 66].

### *3.4.2 Professional Rescue Workers*

Within the group of professional rescue workers, it seems that firefighters have fewer problems compared to emergency healthcare workers and police officers. For example, one study showed that indeed ambulance personnel had more PTSD than firefighters, and also more than police officers [7], while studies in France show that firefighters have much lower PTSD rates than police officers. For example, a year after the 2015 Paris attacks, 3.4% of the firefighters had PTSD, while this was 9.5% among police officers [23]. The same is true after the Oklahoma City Bombing, where firefighters had the lowest PTSD rates of all rescue workers [54, 55]. Some studies also noted specific differences. German studies, for example, showcased that police officers exhibited more aggressive behaviour, while firefighters scored lower on their general quality of life [20, 67].

Clearly, there are also cultural and context related factors at play. For example, 7% of firefighters had PTSD 9 years after 9/11 [68], while 0.3% of the firefighters in Norway had PTSD after not even a year after the Utøya attacks [27]. This might of course be due to the high number of firefighters who died during 9/11, compared to none after Utøya in Norway.

Why, however, would firefighters be much more fit for facing disasters? There are several reasons. First, while paradoxically also a risk factor, is their experience with more disasters. Firefighters will be exposed to many disasters, which provides them with a "framework" and way of working, that can be transposed to all types of disasters—at least to a degree, as 9/11 was a disaster of unparalleled scope at that time. Secondly, as qualitative research shows, firefighters have (1) a quite tight colleague community overall, with firefighters helping each other; (2) often have colleague support systems in place [2, 59, 69]. This is not always the case for rescue workers. For example, a study in Belgium after the 2016 attacks showed that police officers tended to use the mental health issues of others for their own benefits (e.g. promotion) or to dismiss them; in addition, there was no experience with terrorist attacks, nor other large man-made disasters, and as such, no mental health support systems were properly in place or available [69, 70].

## 3.5 Long-Term Mental Health

Studies on mental health in the long term are always rarer than those right after the terrorist attacks. The reason being, often, that academic journals lose interest, and, even more important, there is no financial support for these studies. An additional reason is the difficulty of follow-up: 10 years after an attack, it might be that several of the rescue workers retired, or moved to another job, or passed away, or any other possibility. Thus, longitudinal insights are always limited [71].

Yet, the studies that do exist provide invaluable insights. First, overall, it seems that PTSD does decline to the previous average. Eleven to 13 years after 9/11, 9.7% of the rescue workers still had PTSD [71]. This is high, but below the global expected average of 10% [8, 9]. Similarly, 7% of emergency medical service had PTSD even up to 12 years later, but this is not above average [44].

A year after the 2016 attacks in Nice, a study looked at directly exposed hospital staff: 9.4% had PTSD [72], while 5 years later, this became 8.6% [73]. Studies in Norway show a starker decrease, dropping from 1.3% PTSD 8–11 months after the Norway attacks, to 0.3% [26, 27].

However, overall, despite PTSD being lower, PTSD declined slowly over the years [49], and even up to a decade later, the link between PTSD and terrorism could still be found in some studies [74]. There are few studies that show what show what predicts whether the PTSD that develops would be long-term, though some studies show that anger is a good early indicator of long-term PTSD [75, 76].

## 3.6 Professional Mental Health Aid

Professional mental health aid is, often, quite different among rescue workers compared to the general population. The reason being that rescue workers often have mental health aid present in their workplace, or at least available to contact [2, 25]. However, in general, there is a lot of unmet mental health aid among rescue workers [69, 77].

### *3.6.1 Mental Health Aid*

Qualitative studies have shown that sometimes rescue worker organizations offer aid such as debriefings out of a wish to offer something. In fact, after the attacks in Brussels, among police officers, there was no initial aid, which led to frustration, after which voluntary debriefings were offered, which not everyone followed, which led to more frustration, seemingly because it was not mandatory and therefore some were not able to go to the debriefings [69].

This relates to a more general point found in other studies. Despite the availability of mental health aid programs, rescue workers seldom seek out mental health aid, despite having mental health issues [78]. Some studies suggest that this lack of seeking aid might be related to not knowing about mental health disorders that can arise from disaster exposure [69, 73].

This phenomenon is certainly not related to just terrorism, and is in fact a quite common problem in rescue workers [79]. The reasons for the lack of seeking out aid are stigma, lack of support of colleagues, the retraumatization due to current ongoing work, therapists not being available, fear of showing weakness, and the fear of a breach of confidentiality all hold rescue workers back from seeking out professional help [79, 80]. In terrorism studies, one observation is also that those that had more stress, felt less need to find aid. A possible reason might be, aside from stigma, that these rescue workers recognized the stress as something they had dealt with before [11].

This, then again, is in stark contrast to the aforementioned volunteers and non-professional rescue workers. While professional rescue workers tend to fear consequences for their work if they would seek out mental health aid, volunteers generally do not know where to find mental health aid [81, 82]. This explains why the majority of Red Cross Volunteers did not mental health support receive until 9 months after the January 2015 Paris attacks [60], while after 9/11 volunteers used half as much the health programs on offer compared to professional rescue workers [61], yet volunteers often have a larger need for mental health aid than professionals [81]. This is also seen in qualitative studies. Certain rescue workers would wait months, or up to a year, to seek out mental health care, because they did not want to appear weak. In several cases, the trigger to seek out mental health aid was a severe event, such as flashbacks, aggression, and almost shooting someone. This while non-professionals simply didn't know where to find aid [69].

### *3.6.2 Debriefings*

Debriefings, known under many names, though probably the best-known synonym is "Critical Stress Debriefings," are psychologically aimed discussions with rescue workers after a stressful incident, where they are meant to relive and describe their emotions with regard to the stressful incident [83]. Despite at that point decades of research, COVID-19 papers again pointed to the importance of debriefings for rescue workers [83]. Hence, it is important to again reiterate that psychological debriefings are related to either having no effect, or *causing* PTSD [83, 84]. Furthermore, in addition to their lack of effect or even negative effect, the dissatisfaction with debriefings after terrorism has also been linked with PTSD [85]. However, despite the negative effects, debriefings were common after several terrorist attacks [2, 86, 87]. Studies looking into the effects of these debriefings again show the negative effects of the debriefings [88].

## 3.7 Conclusions and Areas of Attention for Improvement

Rescue workers are at risk of developing mental health issues after disasters. However, in general, the risk is lower among rescue workers than the general population.

One major difference between the general population and rescue workers is that the general population is caught by surprise by disaster, while rescue workers are trained for it. As such, unlike with the general population, there are elements in their preparation that can be improved.

Rescue workers responses are often chaotic, with a lot of difficulties in communicating, and a lot of ad hoc decision making [2, 25]. Some decisions concern life and death, and can be part of future guilt [2]. Hence, better preparation for rescue workers is important [25]. Thus, it remains important to train for mass causality events, because the nature of such events is always different, and training is one of the most important protective factors [1, 89]. Such training can be important for purely practical aspects, such as communication. Communication is key in a disaster setting [89], and yet, is often still an issue in rescue workers [2]. This can even occur simply because of a lack of knowledge of communication devices [89, 90], or unexperienced leadership [91]. Training provides rescue workers with more experience with the disaster plans, teamwork, communication tools, and leadership.

In addition, training for mass causality events teaches general principles that are applicable to all situations. Additionally, it is also important to teach "prioritization" in the acute phase of an attack: what is most important to do in the moment of the rescue [92]. Disaster medicine is, in that sense, radically different, as it operates from the notion that there are limited resources and time, and that people that can be saved, need to be saved first, and those that are seemingly beyond rescue, should not be prioritized [2].

While the response systems towards patients, as in survivors of terrorism, are overall in Western countries quite effective, rescue workers are often left out of the mental health aid response and attention [2, 24]. As one study in England showed, there was a need for psychosocial aid within healthcare staff after the attacks there [25].

## References

1. Wesemann U, Applewhite B, Himmerich H. Investigating the impact of terrorist attacks on the mental health of emergency responders: systematic review. BJPsych Open. 2022;8:e107.
2. Muysewinkel E, Van Deynse H, Van Overmeire R. Comment on 'Posttraumatic stress disorder and depression after the 2018 Strasbourg Christmas Market terrorist attack: a comparison of exposed and non-exposed police personnel': moving towards shared methodology in terrorism-research. Eur J Psychotraumatol. 2023;14:2272476.
3. Giosan C, Malta L, Jayasinghe N, et al. Relationships between memory inconsistency for traumatic events following 9/11 and PTSD in disaster restoration workers. J Anxiety Disord. 2009;23:557–61.
4. Perlman SE, Friedman S, Galea S, et al. Short-term and medium-term health effects of 9/11. Lancet. 2011;378:925–34.
5. Martínez A, Blanch A. Are rescue workers still at risk? A meta-regression analysis of the worldwide prevalence of post-traumatic stress disorder and risk factors. Stress Health. 2024;40:e3372.
6. Berger W, Coutinho ESF, Figueira I, et al. Rescuers at risk: a systematic review and meta-regression analysis of the worldwide current prevalence and correlates of PTSD in rescue workers. Soc Psychiatry Psychiatr Epidemiol. 2012;47:1001–11.
7. Whalley MG, Brewin CR. Mental health following terrorist attacks. Br J Psychiatry. 2007;190:94–6.
8. Paz García-Vera M, Sanz J, Gutiérrez S. A systematic review of the literature on posttraumatic stress disorder in victims of terrorist attacks. Psychol Rep. 2016;119:328–59.
9. Miguel-Tobal JJ, Vindel AC, Iruarrízaga I, et al. Psychopathological repercussions of the March 11 terrorist attacks in Madrid. Psychology Spain; 9.
10. Misra M, Greenberg N, Hutchinson C, et al. Psychological impact upon London Ambulance Service of the 2005 bombings. Occup Med (Lond). 2009;59:428–33.
11. Zimering R, Gulliver SB, Knight J, et al. Posttraumatic stress disorder in disaster relief workers following direct and indirect trauma exposure to Ground Zero. J Trauma Stress. 2006;19:553–7.
12. Stellman JM, Smith RP, Katz CL, et al. Enduring mental health morbidity and social function impairment in World Trade Center rescue, recovery, and cleanup workers: the psychological dimension of an environmental health disaster. Environ Health Perspect. 2008;116:1248–53.
13. Fischer IC, Pietrzak RH, Maercker A, et al. Post-traumatic stress disorder: rethinking diagnosis. Lancet Psychiatry. 2023;10:741–2.
14. Brooks SK, Dunn R, Amlôt R, et al. Social and occupational factors associated with psychological distress and disorder among disaster responders: a systematic review. BMC Psychol. 2016;4:18.

15. Bowler RM, Han H, Gocheva V, et al. Gender differences in probable posttraumatic stress disorder among police responders to the 2001 World Trade Center terrorist attack. Am J Ind Med. 2010;53:1186–96.
16. Whealin JM, Ciro D, Dasaro CR, et al. Race/ethnic differences in prevalence and correlates of posttraumatic stress disorder in World Trade Center responders: results from a population-based, health monitoring cohort. Psychol Trauma. 2022;14:199–208.
17. Ciro D, Pietrzak RH, Lee RJ, et al. Acculturation, coping, and PTSD in Hispanic 9/11 rescue and recovery workers. Psychol Trauma. 2021;13:84–93.
18. Wesemann U, Mahnke M, Polk S, et al. Long-term effects of the terror attack in Berlin in 2016 on paranoid ideation in female emergency personnel. BJPsych Open. 2020;6:e79.
19. Wesemann U, Bühler A, Mahnke M, et al. Longitudinal mental health effects of the 2016 terrorist attack in Berlin on various occupational groups of emergency service personnel. Health Secur. 2020;18:403–8.
20. Wesemann U, Helms C, Polk S, et al. Mistrust among rescue workers after the terrorist attack in Berlin in 2016 – gender-specific health inequality. Disaster Med Public Health Prep. 2023;17:e394.
21. Pollio EW, Wang J, Randle E, et al. A qualitative narrative study of rescue and recovery workers responding to the terrorist bombing of Oklahoma City's Murrah building. J Occup Environ Med. 2024;66:682–8.
22. Motreff Y, Baubet T, Pirard P, et al. Factors associated with PTSD and partial PTSD among first responders following the Paris terror attacks in November 2015. J Psychiatr Res. 2020;121:143–50.
23. Hunt P. Lessons identified from the 2017 Manchester and London terrorism incidents. Part 1: Introduction and the prehospital phase. BMJ Mil Health. 2020;166:111–4.
24. Muysewinkel E, Vesentini L, Van Deynse H, et al. A day in the life: psychological impact on emergency responders during the 22 March 2016 terrorist attacks. Front Psychiatry; 15. Epub ahead of print 12 February 2024. https://doi.org/10.3389/fpsyt.2024.1353130.
25. Skryabina EA, Betts N, Amlôt R, et al. Understanding the psychological impacts of responding to a terrorist incident. Eur J Psychotraumatol; 12. Epub ahead of print 1 January 2021. https://doi.org/10.1080/20008198.2021.1959116.
26. Skogstad L, Fjetland AM, Ekeberg Ø. Exposure and posttraumatic stress symptoms among first responders working in proximity to the terror sites in Norway on July 22, 2011 – a cross-sectional study. Scand J Trauma Resusc Emerg Med. 2015;23:23.
27. Skogstad L, Heir T, Hauff E, et al. Post-traumatic stress among rescue workers after terror attacks in Norway. Occup Med (Chic Ill). 2016;66:528–35.
28. Pedersen MJB, Gjerland A, Rund BR, et al. Emergency preparedness and role clarity among rescue workers during the terror attacks in Norway July 22, 2011. PLoS One. 2016;11:e0156536.
29. Reid BO, Næss-Pleym LE, Bakkelund KE, et al. A cross-sectional study of mental health-, posttraumatic stress symptoms and post exposure changes in Norwegian ambulance personnel. Scand J Trauma Resusc Emerg Med. 2022;30:3.
30. Rubin GJ, Brewin CR, Greenberg N, et al. Psychological and behavioural reactions to the bombings in London on 7 July 2005: cross sectional survey of a representative sample of Londoners. BMJ. 2005;331:606.
31. Wisnivesky JP, Teitelbaum SL, Todd AC, et al. Persistence of multiple illnesses in World Trade Center rescue and recovery workers: a cohort study. Lancet. 2011;378:888–97.
32. Maslow CB, Caramanica K, Welch AE, et al. Trajectories of scores on a screening instrument for PTSD among World Trade Center rescue, recovery, and clean-up workers. J Trauma Stress. 2015;28:198–205.
33. De Stefano C, Orri M, Agostinucci JM, et al. Early psychological impact of Paris terrorist attacks on healthcare emergency staff: a cross-sectional study. Depress Anxiety. 2018;35:275–82.
34. Nourry N, Alsayed Obeid S, Rolling J, et al. Posttraumatic stress disorder and depression after the 2018 Strasbourg Christmas Market terrorist attack: a comparison of exposed and

non-exposed police personnel. Eur J Psychotraumatol; 14. Epub ahead of print 23 November 2023. https://doi.org/10.1080/20008066.2023.2214872.
35. Boffetta P, Hall CB, Todd AC, et al. Cancer risk among World Trade Center rescue and recovery workers: a review. CA Cancer J Clin. 2022;72:308–14.
36. Khalifeh M, Goldfarb DG, Zeig-Owens R, et al. Cancer incidence in World Trade Center rescue and recovery workers by race and ethnicity. Am J Ind Med. 2023;66:1048–55.
37. Li J, Yung J, Qiao B, et al. Cancer incidence in World Trade Center rescue and recovery workers: 14 years of follow-up. J Natl Cancer Inst. 2022;114:210–9.
38. Sigel K, de la Hoz RE, Markowitz SB, et al. Lung cancer incidence among world trade center rescue and recovery workers. Cancer Med. 2022;11:3136–44.
39. Rojano B, West E, Goodman E, et al. Self-management behaviors in World Trade Center rescue and recovery workers with asthma. J Asthma. 2019;56:411–21.
40. Stein CR, Lee DJ, Flamme GA, et al. Persistent post-9/11 hearing problems among World Trade Center Health Registry rescue and recovery workers, 2001 to 2007. J Occup Environ Med. 2017;59:1229–34.
41. Wyka K, Friedman SM, Jordan HT. Probable posttraumatic stress disorder and lower respiratory symptoms among rescue/recovery workers and community members after the 9/11 World Trade Center attacks—a longitudinal mediation analysis. Psychosom Med. 2020;82:115–24.
42. Luft BJ, Schechter C, Kotov R, et al. Exposure, probable PTSD and lower respiratory illness among World Trade Center rescue, recovery and clean-up workers. Psychol Med. 2012;42:1069–79.
43. Liu B, Tarigan LH, Bromet EJ, et al. World Trade Center disaster exposure-related probable posttraumatic stress disorder among responders and civilians: a meta-analysis. PLoS One. 2014;9:e101491.
44. Yip J, Zeig-Owens R, Webber MP, et al. World Trade Center-related physical and mental health burden among New York City Fire Department emergency medical service workers. Occup Environ Med. 2016;73:13–20.
45. Fullerton CS, Ursano RJ, Reeves J, et al. Perceived safety in disaster workers following 9/11. J Nerv Ment Dis. 2006;194:61–3.
46. Razik S, Ehring T, Emmelkamp PMG. Psychological consequences of terrorist attacks: prevalence and predictors of mental health problems in Pakistani emergency responders. Psychiatry Res. 2013;207:80–5.
47. Katz CL, Smith R, Silverton M, et al. Open forum: A mental health program for ground zero rescue and recovery workers: cases and observations. 2006;57:1335–8.
48. Chiu S, Webber MP, Zeig-Owens R, et al. Performance characteristics of the PTSD Checklist in retired firefighters exposed to the World Trade Center disaster. Ann Clin Psychiatry. 2011;23:95–104.
49. Berninger A, Webber MP, Niles JK, et al. Longitudinal study of probable post-traumatic stress disorder in firefighters exposed to the World Trade Center disaster. Am J Ind Med. 2010;53:1177–85.
50. Evans S, Patt I, Giosan C, et al. Disability and posttraumatic stress disorder in disaster relief workers responding to September 11, 2001 World Trade Center disaster. J Clin Psychol. 2009;65:684–94.
51. Luce A, Firth-Cozens J, Midgley S, et al. After the Omagh bomb: posttraumatic stress disorder in health service staff. J Trauma Stress. 2002;15:27–30.
52. Cukor J, Wyka K, Jayasinghe N, et al. Prevalence and predictors of posttraumatic stress symptoms in utility workers deployed to the World Trade Center following the attacks of September 11, 2001. Depress Anxiety. 2011;28:210–7.
53. Bogstrand ST, Skogstad L, Ekeberg Ø. The association between alcohol, medicinal drug use and post-traumatic stress symptoms among Norwegian rescue workers after the 22 July twin terror attacks. Int Emerg Nurs. 2016;28:29–33.
54. North CS, Tivis L, McMillen JC, et al. Coping, functioning, and adjustment of rescue workers after the Oklahoma City bombing. J Trauma Stress. 2002;15:171–5.

55. North CS, Tivis L, McMillen JC, et al. Psychiatric disorders in rescue workers after the Oklahoma City bombing. Am J Psychiatry. 2002;159:857–9.
56. Zvolensky MJ, Farris SG, Kotov R, et al. World Trade Center disaster and sensitization to subsequent life stress: a longitudinal study of disaster responders. Prev Med (Baltim). 2015;75:70–4.
57. Yu S, Brackbill RM, Locke S, et al. Impact of 9/11-related chronic conditions and PTSD comorbidity on early retirement and job loss among World Trade Center disaster rescue and recovery workers. Am J Ind Med. 2016;59:731–41.
58. Pfefferbaum B. The impact of the 1995 Oklahoma City bombing on the partners of firefighters. J Urban Health. 2002;79:364–72.
59. Van Overmeire R, Van Keer R, Bilsen J. Impact of terrorist attacks on social relationships. Clin Psychol Psychother. 2021;28:1472–81.
60. Meudal J, Vandentorren S, Simeoni L, et al. French Red Cross volunteer rescue workers. J Nerv Ment Dis. 2020;208:413–7.
61. Ayers CD, Kehm RD, Cone JE, et al. Disparities in utilization of the World Trade Center Health Program among World Trade Center rescue and recovery workers and volunteers. Int J Environ Res Public Health. 2025;22:643.
62. Feder A, Mota N, Salim R, et al. Risk, coping and PTSD symptom trajectories in World Trade Center responders. J Psychiatr Res. 2016;82:68–79.
63. Pietrzak RH, Feder A, Singh R, et al. Trajectories of PTSD risk and resilience in World Trade Center responders: an 8-year prospective cohort study. Psychol Med. 2014;44:205–19.
64. Zhang G, Pfefferbaum B, Narayanan P, et al. Psychiatric disorders after terrorist bombings among rescue workers and bombing survivors in Nairobi and rescue workers in Oklahoma City. Ann Clin Psychiatry. 2016;28:22–30.
65. Cukor J, Wyka K, Mello B, et al. The longitudinal course of PTSD among disaster workers deployed to the World Trade Center following the attacks of September 11th. J Trauma Stress. 2011;24:506–14.
66. Gjerland A, Pedersen MJB, Ekeberg Ø, et al. Sick-leave and help seeking among rescue workers after the terror attacks in Norway, 2011. Int J Emerg Med. 2015;8:31.
67. Wesemann U, Zimmermann P, Mahnke M, et al. Burdens on emergency responders after a terrorist attack in Berlin. Occup Med (Chic Ill). 2018;68:60–3.
68. Webber MP, Glaser MS, Weakley J, et al. Physician-diagnosed respiratory conditions and mental health symptoms 7–9 years following the World Trade Center disaster. Am J Ind Med. 2011;54:661–71.
69. Van Overmeire R, Muysewinkel E, Van Keer R-L, et al. Victims of the terrorist attacks in Belgium and professional mental health aid barriers: a qualitative study. Front Psychiatry; 12. Epub ahead of print 2 July 2021. https://doi.org/10.3389/fpsyt.2021.638272.
70. Van Overmeire R, Vesentini L, Van Keer R-L, et al. Working experiences of airport employees after a terrorist attack in Belgium: a qualitative study. Int J Disaster Risk Reduct. 2021;64:102515.
71. Bromet EJ, Hobbs MJ, Clouston SAP, et al. DSM-IV post-traumatic stress disorder among World Trade Center responders 11–13 years after the disaster of 11 September 2001 (9/11). Psychol Med. 2016;46:771–83.
72. Bentz L, Vandentorren S, Fabre R, et al. Mental health impact among hospital staff in the aftermath of the Nice 2016 terror attack: the ECHOS de Nice study. BMC Public Health. 2021;21:1372.
73. Prioux C, Marillier M, Vuillermoz C, et al. PTSD and partial PTSD among first responders one and five years after the Paris terror attacks in November 2015. Int J Environ Res Public Health; 20. Epub ahead of print 25 February 2023. https://doi.org/10.3390/ijerph20054160.
74. Soo J, Webber MP, Gustave J, et al. Trends in probable PTSD in firefighters exposed to the World Trade Center disaster, 2001–2010. Disaster Med Public Health Prep. 2011;5:S197–203.

75. Evans S, Giosan C, Patt I, et al. Anger and its association to distress and social/occupational functioning in symptomatic disaster relief workers responding to the September 11, 2001, World Trade Center disaster. J Trauma Stress. 2006;19:147–52.
76. Jayasinghe N, Giosan C, Evans S, et al. Anger and posttraumatic stress disorder in disaster relief workers exposed to the September 11, 2001 World Trade Center disaster. J Nerv Ment Dis. 2008;196:844–6.
77. Jayasinghe N, Spielman L, Cancellare D, et al. Predictors of treatment utilization in world trade center attack disaster workers: role of race/ethnicity and symptom severity. Int J Emerg Ment Health. 2005;7:91–9.
78. Motreff Y, Pirard P, Vuillermoz C, et al. Mental health care utilization by first responders after Paris attacks. Occup Med (Lond). 2022;72:81–90.
79. Jones S, Agud K, McSweeney J. Barriers and facilitators to seeking mental health care among first responders: 'removing the darkness'. J Am Psychiatr Nurses Assoc. 2020;26:43–54.
80. Cogan N, Craig A, Milligan L, et al. 'I've got no PPE to protect my mind': understanding the needs and experiences of first responders exposed to trauma in the workplace. Eur J Psychotraumatol. 2024;15:2395113.
81. Diab O, DePierro J, Cancelmo L, et al. Mental healthcare needs in World Trade Center responders: results from a large, population-based health monitoring cohort. Adm Policy Ment Health Ment Health Serv Res. 2020;47:427–34.
82. DePierro J, Lowe SM, Haugen PT, et al. Mental health stigma and barriers to care in World Trade Center responders: results from a large, population-based health monitoring cohort. Am J Ind Med. 2021;64:208–16.
83. Van Overmeire R. The myth of psychological debriefings during the corona pandemic. J Glob Health; 10. Epub ahead of print December 2020. https://doi.org/10.7189/jogh.10.020344.
84. Mansdorf IJ. Psychological interventions following terrorist attacks. Br Med Bull. 2008;88:7–22.
85. Tran DV, North CS. The association between dissatisfaction with debriefing and post-traumatic stress disorder (PTSD) in rescue and recovery workers for the Oklahoma City bombing. Disaster Med Public Health Prep. 2018;12:718–22.
86. Hammond J, Brooks J. The World Trade Center attack. Helping the helpers: the role of critical incident stress management. Crit Care. 2001;5:315.
87. Kagee A. Concerns about the effectiveness of critical incident stress debriefing in ameliorating stress reactions. Crit Care. 2002;6:88.
88. Wesemann U, Mahnke M, Polk S, et al. Impact of crisis intervention on the mental health status of emergency responders following the Berlin terrorist attack in 2016. Disaster Med Public Health Prep. 2020;14:168–72.
89. Craigie RJ, Farrelly PJ, Santos R, et al. Manchester Arena bombing: lessons learnt from a mass casualty incident. BMJ Mil Health. 2020;166:72–5.
90. De Cauwer H, Barten D, Willems M, et al. Communication failure in the prehospital response to major terrorist attacks: lessons learned and future directions. Eur J Trauma Emerg Surg. 2023;49:1741–50.
91. Brooks SK, Dunn R, Sage CAM, et al. Risk and resilience factors affecting the psychological wellbeing of individuals deployed in humanitarian relief roles after a disaster. J Ment Health. 2015;24:385–413.
92. Obiajulu J, DeSoucy E, Robb D, et al. Lessons learned from a large-scale military mass casualty incident: reevaluation of the response to the Khobar Towers bombing. Mil Med. 2025;190:122–4.

# Chapter 4
# Watch Out: A Public Health Perspective on the Societal Impact of Terrorism

## 4.1 Introduction

Terrorism, other than crime or interpersonal violence, can have an impact on society at large. If terrorism has as aim to create fear, to cause change in societies, etc. [1], then it is of the upmost importance for public health sciences to investigate whether it succeeds, and to see what it in fact affects.

Most forms of evidence for this link come from either survey studies on media watching of terrorist attacks, or through administrative data showcasing an increase (or decrease) of certain diseases linked with stress reactions.

The chapter is divided into three main parts.

First, the link between media watching and mental health issues is discussed. Secondly, administrative data on mental health after terrorist attacks is investigated. Three, data that indicates behavioural changes and opinion changes in the population.

The link between these three parts is on the hand is the indirect exposure of terrorism on the population at large. Furthermore, while the first part is explicitly about media watching, the second and third part on administrative data and other data is probably also mostly caused by media watching.

---

Passages in this chapter are based on my doctoral thesis, defended in 2021. Van Overmeire, R. (2021). The association between exposure to terrorist attacks and mental health in Belgium. [PhD Thesis, Vrije Universiteit Brussel]. VUB Press. https://cris.vub.be/ws/portalfiles/portal/86873200/1_PDFsam_Van_Overmeire_Roel_PhD_thesis_20.12.2021.pdf



R. Van Overmeire, *Terrorism, Mental Health and Aftercare*,
https://doi.org/10.1007/978-3-032-31560-1_4

## 4.2 Media Watching and Mental Health

### *4.2.1 Media Watching of Terrorist Attacks Among the General Population*

What in this chapter is called "media watching" refers to the watching of images or reports concerning terrorist attacks, either through television, radio, the internet… What is specific about this type of media watching, is that after a terrorist attack news media will generally broadcast 24 h non-stop about the event [2]. Thus, this allows people to view the aftermath of the attacks, and often events unfolding, in real time.

Several studies have stated to have found a relation between media watching and mental health issues among indirectly exposed people (e.g. people who only viewed an attack through media) [3–10]. Mental health issues include post-traumatic stress disorder (PTSD) symptoms, depression symptoms, anxiety symptoms, insomnia, the content of dreams, and somatic symptoms [4, 11–14].

### *4.2.2 The Hours of Watching*

It seems that the most important indicator in this relationship is the number of hours of watching media related to terrorism. One study, 1–3 weeks after 9/11, showed that watching more than 4 h of reports on the terrorist attacks, predicted mental health issues 2–3 years later [15]. Another important indicator is the identification with the victims. Studies after the sniper attacks in Washington D.C. in 2002, showed that the more a viewer identified with the victims of the sniper attacks, the more chance for mental health issues [16–18].

### *4.2.3 Proximity*

Naturally, what plays a role as well, is proximity. This means in the case of the general population: how close is someone living or working nearby the attacks? For example, in 2004, bombings of trains caused 191 deaths in Madrid, Spain. One study, 1–3 months after these attacks, looked at the role of proximity in a general population of Madrid: how close to the place of these bombing did respondents work or live? It showed that 2.3% had PTSD and 8% had depression symptoms, while those living closest to the site of the attacks had even higher PTSD symptoms (4.3%) [19].

However, another study, on the 2016 attacks in Belgium, showed that if the number of hours goes beyond 3 h of watching a day, it has the same effect as living or working nearby the place of the attacks [4]. This is a similar result to studies after the Boston Marathon Bombing, where watching more than 6 h of terrorism related media content caused more acute stress than being directly exposed [20]. Thus, this would mean that media watching can be just as impactful as simply living nearby and that people living far away from a terrorist attack would develop mental health issues, despite the distance [21].

### 4.2.4 Content of Media

Yet, the relation is more complicated. First, there is the content of the media as well. For example, media reports on mass violence that are overtly negative and affective tend to affect people more, and create a higher perception of threat [22, 23]. This perception of terrorist threat is very much linked with mental health issues [12]. In one study, more than 5 years after 9/11, PTSD symptoms still were associated with a greater worry of future terrorist attacks [23], which was also seen in a study years after the Belgian attacks [24].

### 4.2.5 Prior Traumatization

Secondly, an additional predictor for the effect of media watching of terrorism on mental health is prior traumatization (e.g. having been exposed to trauma before a terrorist attack) [20, 25]. Studies show that prior exposure to large scale community events seems to be linked with a higher vulnerability to effects of media reports on terrorism [8, 20, 26, 27].

### 4.2.6 Feedback Effect

In fact, there seems to be a feedback effect in media watching. As mentioned, sensational media reports can increase the perception of terrorist threat, which in itself is linked with more mental health issues [12, 28]. However, people with more mental health issues will generally also watch more media about terrorist attacks [29]. That indicates therefore that there is vicious cycle, where mental health issues get worse with watching terrorist attacks, and terrorist attacks seem to make mental health issues worse [4, 30].

Another study after the Washington sniper attacks seems to suggest that while feeling unsafe is linked with media watching and mental health issues, it might be that the feeling of unsafety was already there and then enhanced by the sniper attacks [31]. This indicates yet another feedback effect, where cause and effect are difficult to estimate: what came first, a cause for unsafety or the feeling of unsafety?

**New Media**

New media forms, such as social media, affect the relationship as well as television.

In fact, at first sight, it seems to do this even more [2]. Both television viewing as well as online news viewing were both correlated with more graphic content of terrorist attacks [2]. Naturally, many studies investigate the negative effects of social media on youth and people, but the overwhelming majority of studies on media watching of terrorism and mental health are based on watching television.

### *4.2.7 Media Watching of Terrorist Attacks Among Indirectly Exposed Children and Adolescents*

While direct exposure is a more important indicator for children's and adolescents' mental health issues after terrorist attacks, media contact fulfills that role among those indirectly exposed [32–34]. Those most vulnerable to experience high stress symptoms among indirectly exposed children are 10- to 13-year-olds, girls, minorities, children with a lower-socioeconomic status, children living close to the place of attacks and those with prior trauma [35–37].

Several studies show an increase in post-traumatic stress symptoms and other mental health issues among children and adolescents due to media watching of terrorist attacks [36–39]. For example, studies after the Paris attack of 13/11/2015 showed that youth get more anxiety, depression, and are emotionally dysregulated due to watching too much info on social networks [40], which is similar to findings after the Boston Marathon Bombing [41]. Children who lived in Boston during the bombing, and who watched more than 3 h of media on the manhunt on the perpetrators, tended to have more post-traumatic stress symptoms, but also conduct problems [42]. Similarly, after the Oklahoma City Bombing, school children kept experiencing mental health reactions to the coverage of the attacks [33, 43].

This relationship between media watching and mental health issues for children and adolescents is found around the world. Studies have shown that even in London or India there was an increase in stress among children after 9/11, despite the distance [44, 45]. After the 2015 Paris attacks and the 2016 Belgium attacks, Italian students experienced stress reactions [46], while a relation between news coverage of the bombing and mental health issues were found among school children even 100 miles away from Oklahoma [47].

Additionally, children are often dependent on the reactions of their parents [48, 49], though children might also affect the reactions of their parents [34]. This means that parents who show fear and anxiety to the attacks might cause fear in their children, while this also holds true vice versa.

As mentioned, prior traumatization is a risk factor, and so is having mental disorders before the attacks. Children who already had mental disorders before the attacks often had an increase in symptoms through watching terrorist attacks on television [50].

Terrorist attacks also disrupt routines, which is also linked with more mental health issues. After the sniper attacks in Washington, daily routines were disrupted, and the more disrupted they were, the more issues children seemed to have [51].

The sensational way of covering attacks, without any context for children, might affect the way they view the world and increase their perception of the likelihood of not just terrorist attacks, but also other forms of disasters[52, 53]. One example provided by Atwood and Donnelly [54] is that children between the ages of 7 and 11 did not know the difference between a Muslim neighbour and a Muslim terrorist.

Indirectly exposed children will often get less contextualization for attacks [47, 55, 56]. This uncertainty about the attacks can make children fantasize about the attacks in such a way that they make it worse than it is. For example, in one qualitative study, a 13-year-old girl wondered

> Do we have a chance on World War 3? [57]

While in the same study, another wondered:

> Should I be afraid of the IS? Can they attack our (town) or do we have enough soldiers to make sure they don't come here anymore? [57]

While schools and teachers can generally give guidance [58], it seems that teachers themselves are not always prepared to give those answers [57]. This should not be too surprising considering the previous parts: teachers are also affected by terrorist attacks and thus might also have difficulty coping immediately after attacks [37].

### 4.2.8 Media Watching Among Directly Exposed People

In general, media watching is a poor direct predictor of mental health issues for those directly exposed (e.g. survivors of attacks) [33, 59, 60], also among directly exposed children [33, 34]. However, the role of media watching is more subtle. A longitudinal study after the 2013 Boston Marathon bombings collected data of survivors of the bombing, and again of those survivors 5 days after the Pulse Nightclub Massacre (roughly 3 years after the Boston Marathon Bombings). The study showed that the mental health issues affected the perception of future negative events, which in turn was related with more media consumption, and more stress after the Pulse Nightclub Massacre [30]. In other words: media watching of terrorism related violence is linked with mental health issues, which in turn lead to more media watching [30]. This would explain why some studies [59] do not see a link among directly exposed people between mental health and media watching, because the link is indirect, and not a direct link.

**Media Consumption Among Indirectly and Directly Exposed People**
While among indirectly exposed people, the principle of more hours of watching terrorism related media leading to a higher chance of developing mental health problems holds, among survivors of a previous terrorist attack, avoidance of media on new attacks can be observed. One study showed that some Oklahoma City Bombing survivors would discontinue watching 9/11 media due to fear [6], while in Belgium, qualitative studies show a split image: either survivors would avoid everything related to new terrorist attacks, or obsessively investigate all information available about new attacks [61, 62].

### *4.2.9 Criticism*

Studies on the link between media watching and terrorism have garnered criticism, as there are many factors that come in to play in the relation between media watching of violence and mental health, such as cultural factors, social factors, etc. [63]. As Durodié and Wainwright [63] state, such studies "*posit a low view of the public's ability to think critically.*"

Another problem of these types of studies is that many were often performed long after the attack, while asking participants to recall how much terrorism related media they watched after the attacks [4]. There are only a few studies that actually took place either a week to a few months after the initial attack [4, 64]. This lag in surveying responses is problematic for the simple reason that

1. There is recall bias. It is difficult for people to recall how much of the news they watched after an attack if this asked long after. One study, for example, was performed 35 months (almost 3 years) later [65].
2. Related to this, is that people who perceive that the terrorist attacks had a severe impact on their mental health, and who have suffered from anxiety issues, might overestimate their media watching, while people for whom it was not as impactful, might underestimate their media watching. As studies have shown, people with mental health issues already view more media [29]. In other words: the results might be getting skewed, which would result in creating the illusion that a lot of media watching creates more mental health issues, simply because the reporting of the hours of media watching is higher among people whom it affected, yet it might also be high among those whom it did not affect, but who simply underreport it [4].

Additionally, people living far away from attack sites might relate their issues to the attacks [10, 38, 66], but that does not mean that these attacks actually caused those mental health symptoms. For example, a person who had severe mental health issues before the attacks, might "use" a terrorist attack as a specific cause and origin for their mental health issues. Such biases and narratives can come in many forms, whether as hind-sight bias, or illness narratives that explain the condition due to a specific event [67, 68]. Similarly, attribution theory shows that people tend to need such explanations for how things are: X caused Y, even when Y came before X [69, 70]. In fact, as Chap. 9 shows, survivors of terrorist attacks need for recognition is partly driven by a need to show that their mental health symptoms were done to them by perpetrators [71]. Related to this, one could argue that due to the need to attribute their mental health symptoms to something, and due to respondents perhaps knowing what a researcher is looking for, respondents might complete a questionnaire in such a way that their own attribution of X to Y (when Y came before X) makes sense in the questionnaire [72].

Following this, another problem of these studies are the weak research designs, which are often cross-sectional, meaning: one-time measurements. Such design eliminates any possibility of causal explanations, meaning: media watching *causing* mental health symptoms is impossible to prove [5]. Therefore, the issue of causation (or more accurate: the absence of it) is quite limiting of the interpretation of such studies [73, 74].

**Type of Media**

When discussing "media watching of terrorism," there are still major differences between countries that are difficult to take into account. In fact, most of these studies are about 9/11 or other U.S.-based terrorist attacks. With a few exceptions, the USA is the only country that has published so much on the link between media watching of terrorist attacks and mental health.

This is a limitation for any form of generalization because the USA has a completely different form of media. The 24/7 news media are simply not as popular in other countries as they are in the USA.

Furthermore, as the majority of studies are based on 9/11, it seems as if the majority of our knowledge on the link comes from an attack that is the biggest terrorist attack of all. The attacks were such a sui generis attack, that it might skew findings—after all, while the Boston Marathon bombing could be compared with for example the bombings of the public transport in London or Brussels or Madrid, 9/11 was and still is unprecedented. The consequences, both emotionally, mentally and politically, are not comparable with other terrorist attacks. This holds true however for almost all terrorist attacks. For example, one cannot compare the October 7th attack in Israel with any other attack, due to its scale, but also its context.

Additionally, the *Diagnostic and Statistical Manual of Mental Disorders-5* (DSM-5) removed media-watching as inclusion for PTSD, as the relation between viewing an event through media and developing PTSD symptoms was difficult to properly explain from a psychiatric viewpoint. For example, it is unclear how a typical reaction to stress, such as a fight-or-flight response, would be caused with just images and not a direct threat. However, that does not mean using PTSD in media watching studies is useless. In fact, there are still studies on media-watching of terrorism and PTSD [65]. These studies often use DSM-IV definitions, as they are longitudinal and often were started before the DSM-5 change [75].

**Terrorism as Trauma or Something Else?**

When measuring PTSD, symptoms often need to be "attributed" to something. Many studies do not do this, and simply assume any PTSD is due to terrorism [63]. However, when looking beyond the assumed relation between terrorism and mental health issues—thus, looking at other forms of trauma as explanation for mental health issues—the relation becomes much weaker. For example, one study on media watching and 9/11 showed that indeed, 9/11 was not the biggest explanation for the mental health issues of people whose issues would otherwise be assumed to be the cause [76]. In fact, when viewing only those who viewed 9/11 as the worst trauma, despite it being an indirect exposure through for example media, only 0.3% had PTSD [76]. This is of course logical: if people experienced other traumatic events in person (e.g. violence, robbery, sexual assault), then this direct exposure will probably have a much bigger impact than an indirect exposure—even when this is 9/11, while if the indirect exposure of 9/11 is the worst event, it might be that these people had no prior trauma exposure, meaning their risk for PTSD was already lower. This is also no doubt why, as seen throughout this chapter, prior traumatization was a risk factor: because media watching of terrorism might increase mental health issues, but will very seldom actually cause them.

Additionally, some studies suggest that there is actual possibility for post-traumatic growth in the population after such attacks [77], which indicates that there are other links possible with media watching after terrorism, including positive ones.

Thus, there is reason to doubt the link between media watching of mass trauma and mental health in general. One review, for example, showed that the link between mass trauma and depression in children is indeed inconclusive based on a wealthy of evidence [59].

## 4.3 Relation Between Terrorism and Health in the General Population

Administrative data shows a possible short-term impact of terrorism on public health. Often these are (probably) caused by stress reactions, and many of these observations are high level, meaning that it is difficult to estimate in what way they are coincidence or not. It seems overall that there is reason to assume an "impact" on the population at large, though, as always, how much of it is truly due to the terrorist attacks will depend on the size of the attack, timing, context, and other factors.

### 4.3.1 *Ischemic Heart Diseases*

Terrorist attacks can be associated with more somatic issues in the general population [4]. For example, higher rates of ischemic heart diseases due the emotional stress are more likely to be found after terrorist attacks [75, 78]. Somatic reactions were noticed as well in children. One small sample showed that children who had experienced the severe stress of 9/11 had temporally more severe cardiac output responses under stress [79].

After 9/11, several studies showed that there were more heart attacks nationwide—even in places not under any threat of attack at that point [80–83]. After the 2011 Norway attacks, a similar observation was found, where an increase of 5% in heart attacks was found in the first 4 weeks [84], yet, in France, this observation between heart attacks and terrorist attacks was not found [85].

### 4.3.2 *Pregnancy Outcomes*

The two main issues related to terrorism and pregnancy are pre-term births, and a low birthweight in the short term. One study after 9/11 showed more births after the attacks, similarly to an increase in birth after the 2016 Norway attacks, though the number of pre-term births was only moderate, and in New York itself, there was an increased chance of lower birth weight in the months after the attacks [84, 86].

Another study showed a more nuanced view, where the effect of 9/11 on lower birth weights and pre-term births was not seen in New York or among Arab Americans (who generally do have more issues than the general population) [87], though lower birth weights and pre-terms births were observed in Spain after the 2004 Madrid attacks. Then again, there was more infant mortality in New York after 9/11, which wasn't found in Spain after the 2004 attacks [88]. In short, as with ischemic heart diseases: sometimes it is observed after terrorist attacks, sometimes not.

### 4.3.3 *Mental Health Data*

Other administrative data suggest an increase in stress related disorders. For example, a study in Denmark showed such an increase after the 9/11 attacks [89]. Interestingly, the increase in these disorders was even larger after the Utøya attacks in Norway [90]. It is hypnotized that this is due to the proximity [89]. Similarly, psychiatric patients in the USA also exhibit higher PTSD symptoms after 9/11 [91], while after the 2016 attacks in Norway, there was an increase in hospitalizations for schizophrenia or psychosis for 4 weeks [84]. One study in France also showed an increase in benzodiazepine usage after the terrorist attacks, possibly due to sleeping issues [92].

These data suggest something noted earlier: people with mental health disorders prior to the attacks seem to have a higher risk of having more mental health issues after the attacks.

### *4.3.4 Suicide*

A meta-analysis of different forms of disasters and mass-causality events found a higher suicidal ideation and suicide attempts, especially among women [93], but in the case of actual suicide, studies on terrorism are conflicting.

In a study that looked at 2 years before and 2 years after 9/11, an increase in suicide attempts was found [94], while a study in New York after 9/11 found no change in suicide rates [95], even though another found a decrease in rate [96]. Abroad, suicide rates went up in the Netherlands after 9/11 [97], while in Germany no such change was found [98], and in England and Wales researchers even found a decrease [99]. After the attacks in Belgium 2016, the suicide rates didn't change. However, interestingly, suicide doubled in Belgium after the Paris attacks in 2015. This increase lasted 2 weeks, which was the period that Brussels was put on the highest alert level, and the suicide numbers dropped together with the lowering of the highest alert level [100]. Similarly, the number of suicides after the 2016 Norway attacks increased with 105% the first week after the attacks, and 45% for the first 4 weeks [84]. Finally, after 9/11, there was an increase in aircraft assisted pilot suicides [101].

The theory of suicide by the sociologist Émile Durkheim is one of the most famous ways of explaining suicide in society [102]. Over more than 100 years ago he found that suicide has social explanations, not just individual reasons and can therefore be correlated with external threat that affect society, such as war. However, this is not always a negative impact, as external threats can actually cause suicide rates to drop [75, 102]. Based on this idea, some researchers suspect that there will be more social cohesion and even post-traumatic growth in society due to external threats [77], and also that suicide rates will go down [97–99].

There are a couple of reasons this theory does not hold up for terrorism, though. First, the assumption that terrorism leads to a higher sense of solidarity within the nation, is arguable from a theoretical standpoint, as Durkheim never explicitly stated that terrorism has this effect; of course, also because terrorism as such was not defined as it is now [102]. The assumption that a decrease should be found for terrorism is based on an ambiguous reading of Durkheim, where "war" is equated to "terrorism."

The lens of economic failing is another way of looking at the issue, as Durkheim found that suicide increase during economic difficult periods [102, 103]. Indeed, as shown later in this chapter, due to tourism dropping, there is a clear impact of terrorism on the economy, yet what way the quick economic pressure would take its toll on suicide rates is unclear.

In fact, what Durkheim calls “anomic” suicides coincides with the increase of the threat levels in Belgium after the Paris-attacks, or with the Patriot Act measures taken by the U.S. government after the 9/11 attacks. These types of suicides occur during times of extreme stress or pressure in society, and when society is perceived to have changed for the worst [102]. That might be the most fitting, and satisfying, explanation, as this fits both suicide during economic downfall, as well as the restriction after attacks [75].

It does seem based on the findings, that either way there is no way to generalize the finding that suicide should decrease.

Finally, one can argue that most of these studies on suicide suffer from methodological issues that are inherent to studying suicide. Sometimes the samples are small (e.g. in the case of Belgium), but mostly the issue is that there is no way to connect a population event with a suicide.

That being said, the phenomenon of suicide due to societal events is notable in other contexts as well. For example, there is the Werther effect, which is the idea that people might commit suicide in a form of imitation of the death a celebrity [104]. For example, after the suicide of comedian Robin Williams, famous for Good Will Hunting, suicides increased 10% [105]. While overall there indeed seems to be more suicide after a celebrity suicide [106], this is case where it will depend on one celebrity to the other. It is therefore no golden rule; in fact, the origin of the Werther effect comes from the book by Von Goethe, in which the main character commits suicide, which had supposedly led to a Europe wide spread of imitations. Ironically, considering the origin of the name “Werther effect,” this is a myth, as there is no evidence of a widespread increase in suicide after the publication and success of the book [107].

## 4.4 Terrorist Attacks and Behaviour and Opinions of the Population

### *4.4.1 Opinions and Outlook on Society*

Studies after 9/11 showed that 22% of the general population in the USA viewed it as their worst life experience, even years afterwards [108]. Indeed, studies show that indeed, terrorism seems to leave its mark on society at large, but often in ways that are more related to our opinions or behavior.

People who have a high perception of new terrorist attacks tend to have more support for military interventions [109], a more negative worldview [110], a greater trust in the government [38], have changed opinions about migration [111], are less forgiving [112], and have changed political believes [113] and support what would otherwise they would have otherwise seen as unjust measures [114, 115]. As one study suggests, the underlying mechanism for these opinions is fear [116].

Mental health issues are also linked with more racism among non-directly exposed people [117]. In fact, watching news reports on suicide bombers that do not follow media guidelines tended to increase the islamophobia of those watching it [118]. Indeed, especially Muslims felt singled out after the 9/11 and the London terrorist attacks and had more mental health issues [119, 120].

While in the USA, terrorist attacks increased distrust of Muslim Americans [121], after the Christchurch attacks, there was actually more trust in Muslim Americans, who were the target of those attacks [122]. Within the Muslim community, while there was more terrorism anxiety, there was also a greater sense of community, and no change in the general wellbeing or psychological distress [123]. In other words, societal outlooks were changed, not the mental health [123].

Thus, opinions and societal views seem to get affected among those who view the likelihood of more terrorist attacks to be large.

### 4.4.2 Behaviour

In addition to this, behavior changes are also seemingly correlated with terrorism. For example, after 9/11, there was a decrease in air travel, and an increase in transport through car in the USA [124].. In fact, the airline industry suffered more financial losses in 2001 and 2002 than the entirety of profits between 1955 and 2000 [125].

The changed transport behaviour in society is also noticeable in other countries. Over half a year after the London bombings, there was fewer public transport and a decreased intent to travel, even though the mental health consequences for the population seemed to dissipate [110, 120, 126, 127].

A study, 2.5 years after the attacks in Belgium, seems to indicate that while the mental health symptoms themselves became less severe in the Brussels population, the population had adjusted their habits of transportation (the attacks were on the metro and the airport), avoiding large squares more, taking public transport less, etc. [24], while after the Washington sniper attacks, almost half of a sample went less to parks and public spaces [128].

It could be that terrorism has an impact on behavioural changes related to the nature of the terrorist attack. For example, attacks on public transport led to avoidance of that public transport, while attacks with planes lead to avoidance of planes, and attacks on open spaces lead to the avoidance of parks and other areas.

In a more indirect way, the possible behavioural impact might be seen in the Boston marathon bombings and the subsequent manhunt. During and after this manhunt, there was an increase of violence in the youth of Boston [129].

One clear exception to behavioural changes seems to be alcohol abuse or drug abuse. For example, despite at first seemingly evidence that drug use increased among already active drug users in the New York state area after 9/11, there is more evidence that it did in fact not [130, 131].

### *4.4.3 The Economy*

The economy also seems to be affected by terrorism, though mainly due to tourism related factors. For example, after the Belgium terrorist attacks, national statistics show a severe impact on the economy in Belgium, due to less tourism [132], which had also been observed after 9/11 [133]. Similarly, after the sniper attacks in Washington in 2002, consumer confidence suffered a dip [134], and as mentioned, the airline industry suffered gigantic financial losses after 9/11 [125].

Similarly, overall, terrorist threat has a relationship with the perception of the financial markets—the markets become more sensitive [135]. Naturally, this is not dissimilar with war or any other major event (e.g. the dip in the market during the first months of the covid pandemic).

Less studied is the relationship between these financial issues in society and the consequences for the mental health of the population. One study showed that around 7% schoolchildren up north of the WTC-attacks showed PTSD symptoms 8 months after 9/11, but these symptoms were mainly linked with financial difficulties due to 9/11, not due to 9/11 itself [136].

## 4.5 Summary

In short, there is evidence that terrorism affects the population of a country, and even outside the country that suffers from a terrorist attack. This impact can be acute, but does not seem to cause chronic issues. The main group that is affected by indirect exposure might actually be those who already suffer from problems, whether it is a weak heart, mental disorders, or suicidal thoughts. Terrorist attacks might in fact "push" them towards a heart attack, more mental health issues or suicide.

Aside from the stress impact, terrorism does reach, partly, its goal of achieving changes in society: it can extremism and fear in a population, and can have real economic consequences. While certainly a lot of this behaviour fades after years go by, it seems the impact of terrorism on society is not of a significant mental health nature, but a behavioural one that is not measured in mental health questionnaires.

Policy makers should therefore be aware of this impact, and can work on providing teachers support to contextualise terrorist attacks to children. Additionally, policy can give messages of hope and support to the population to avoid those with suicidal thoughts to act on them. Other than that, terrorism might be a storm that society has to pass through, but like all storms, it passes.

## References


1. Schmid AP. Defining terrorism. 2023.
2. Jones NM, Garfin DR, Holman EA, et al. Media use and exposure to graphic content in the week following the Boston Marathon bombings. Am J Community Psychol. 2016;58:47–59.
3. Pfefferbaum B, Palka J, North CS. Media contact and posttraumatic stress in employees of New York City area businesses after the September 11 attacks. Disaster Med Public Health Prep. 2022;16:163–9.
4. Van Overmeire R, Stene LE, Vandekerckhove M, et al. Threat through the screen? Association between proximity and/or watching media coverage of a terrorist attack and health. Int J Environ Res Public Health. 2023;20:2876.
5. Pfefferbaum B, Tucker P, Pfefferbaum RL, et al. Media effects in youth exposed to terrorist incidents: a historical perspective. Curr Psychiatry Rep. 2018;20:11.
6. Pfefferbaum B, Nitiéma P, Pfefferbaum RL, et al. Reactions of Oklahoma City bombing survivors to media coverage of the September 11, 2001, attacks. Compr Psychiatry. 2016;65:70–8.
7. Ahern J, Galea S, Resnick H, et al. Television images and psychological symptoms after the September 11 terrorist attacks. Psychiatry Interpers Biolog Processes. 2002;65:289–300.
8. Garfin DR, Holman EA, Silver RC. Exposure to prior negative life events and responses to the Boston marathon bombings. Psychol Trauma. 2020;12:320–9.
9. Stickley A, Oh H, Sumiyoshi T, et al. The September 11, 2001, terrorist attacks, media exposure, and psychotic experiences among Asian and Latino Americans. Psychiatry Clin Neurosci. 2020;74:572–3.
10. Ford JD, Adams ML, Dailey WF. Factors associated with receiving help and risk factors for disaster-related distress among Connecticut adults 5–15 months after the September 11th terrorist incidents. Soc Psychiatry Psychiatr Epidemiol. 2006;41:261–70.
11. Goodwin R, Lemola S, Ben-Ezra M. Media use and insomnia after terror attacks in France. J Psychiatr Res. 2018;98:47–50.
12. Deschepper R, Six S, Gidron Y, et al. Association between feeling threatened by a terrorist attack and subjective health: a web survey a week after the attacks of 22 March 2016 in Belgium. Eur J Psychotraumatol; 9. Epub ahead of print 1 January 2018. https://doi.org/10.1080/20008198.2018.1500821.
13. Propper RE, Stickgold R, Keeley R, et al. Is television traumatic?: Dreams, stress, and media exposure in the aftermath of September 11, 2001. Psychol Sci. 2007;18:334–40.
14. Bulkeley K, Kahan TL. The impact of September 11 on dreaming. Conscious Cogn. 2008;17:1248–56.
15. Silver RC, Holman EA, Andersen JP, et al. Mental- and physical-health effects of acute exposure to media images of the September 11, 2001, attacks and the Iraq war. Psychol Sci. 2013;24:1623–34.
16. Herberman Mash HB, Ursano RJ, Benevides KN, et al. Identification with terrorist victims of the Washington, DC sniper attacks: posttraumatic stress and depression. J Trauma Stress. 2016;29:41–8.
17. Mash PHBH, Fullerton PCS, Ursano MRJ. Post-traumatic stress symptoms following sniper attacks: effects of television viewing and identification with victims. Am J Disaster Med. 2018;13:29–36.
18. Mash HBH, Fullerton CS, Benevides KN, et al. Identification with terrorist attack victims: association with television viewing and prior life threat. Disaster Med Public Health Prep. 2018;12:337–44.
19. Miguel-Tobal JJ, Cano-Vindel A, Gonzalez-Ordi H, et al. PTSD and depression after the Madrid March 11 train bombings. J Trauma Stress. 2006;19:69–80.
20. Holman EA, Garfin DR, Silver RC. Media's role in broadcasting acute stress following the Boston Marathon bombings. Proc Natl Acad Sci. 2014;111:93–8.

21. Blanchard EB, Rowell D, Kuhn E, et al. Posttraumatic stress and depressive symptoms in a college population one year after the September 11 attacks: the effect of proximity. Behav Res Ther. 2005;43:143–50.
22. Wormwood JB, Lin Y-R, Lynn SK, et al. Correction: Psychological impact of mass violence depends on affective tone of media content. PLoS One. 2021;16:e0250756.
23. Garfin DR, Poulin MJ, Blum S, et al. Aftermath of terror: a nationwide longitudinal study of posttraumatic stress and worry across the decade following the September 11, 2001 terrorist attacks. J Trauma Stress. 2018;31:146–56.
24. Van Overmeire R, Six S, Deschepper R, et al. Association between feeling threatened, behaviour and symptoms of anxiety and depression: two and a half years after the terrorist attacks in Belgium. Community Ment Health J. 2022;58:657–65.
25. Piwowarczyk L, Rous D, Mancuso A, et al. Impact of the Boston Marathon bombing and its aftermath on refugees and survivors of torture. J Immigr Minor Health. 2016;18:764–70.
26. Garfin DR, Holman EA, Silver RC. Cumulative exposure to prior collective trauma and acute stress responses to the Boston Marathon bombings. Psychol Sci. 2015;26:675–83.
27. Busso DS, McLaughlin KA, Sheridan MA. MEDIA EXPOSURE AND SYMPATHETIC NERVOUS SYSTEM REACTIVITY PREDICT PTSD SYMPTOMS AFTER THE BOSTON MARATHON BOMBINGS. Depress Anxiety. 2014;31:551–8.
28. Rubaltelli E, Scrimin S, Moscardino U, et al. Media exposure to terrorism and people's risk perception: the role of environmental sensitivity and psychophysiological response to stress. Br J Psychol. 2018;109:656–73.
29. de Wit L, van Straten A, Lamers F, et al. Are sedentary television watching and computer use behaviors associated with anxiety and depressive disorders? Psychiatry Res. 2011;186:239–43.
30. Thompson RR, Jones NM, Holman EA, et al. Media exposure to mass violence events can fuel a cycle of distress. Sci Adv; 5. Epub ahead of print 5 April 2019. https://doi.org/10.1126/sciadv.aav3502.
31. Fullerton CS, Mash HBH, Morganstein JC, et al. Active shooter and terrorist event-related posttraumatic stress and depression: television viewing and perceived safety. Disaster Med Public Health Prep. 2019;13:570–6.
32. Duarte CS, Wu P, Cheung A, et al. Media use by children and adolescents from New York City 6 months after the WTC attack. J Trauma Stress. 2011;24:553–6.
33. Pfefferbaum B. Children's exposure to single incidents of terrorism: perspectives over 25 years since the Oklahoma City bombing. Curr Psychiatry Rep. 2020;22:39.
34. Pfefferbaum B, North CS. The association between parent-reported child disaster reactions and posttraumatic stress disorder in parent survivors of disasters and terrorism. Ann Clin Psychiatry. 2020;32:256–65.
35. Becker-Blease KA, Finkelhor D, Turner H. Media exposure predicts children's reactions to crime and terrorism. J Trauma Dissoc. 2008;9:225–48.
36. Lengua LJ, Long AC, Smith KI, et al. Pre-attack symptomatology and temperament as predictors of children's responses to the September 11 terrorist attacks. J Child Psychol Psychiatry. 2005;46:631–45.
37. Noppe IC, Noppe LD, Bartell D. Terrorism and resilience: adolescents' and teachers' responses to September 11, 2001. Death Stud. 2006;30:41–60.
38. Ford CA, Udry JR, Gleiter K, et al. Reactions of young adults to September 11, 2001. Arch Pediatr Adolesc Med. 2003;157:572.
39. Kennedy C, Charlesworth A, Chen J-L. Disaster at a distance: impact of 9.11.01 televised news coverage on mothers' and children's health. J Pediatr Nurs. 2004;19:329–39.
40. Monfort E, Afzali MH. Traumatic stress symptoms after the November 13th 2015 terrorist attacks among young adults: the relation to media and emotion regulation. Compr Psychiatry. 2017;75:68–74.

41. Comer JS, DeSerisy M, Greif Green J. Caregiver-reports of internet exposure and posttraumatic stress among Boston-area youth following the 2013 Marathon bombing. Evid-Based Pract Child Adolesc Mental Health. 2016;1:86–102.
42. Comer JS, Dantowitz A, Chou T, et al. Adjustment among area youth after the Boston Marathon bombing and subsequent manhunt. Pediatrics. 2014;134:7–14.
43. Pfefferbaum B, Nixon SJ, Tivis RD, et al. Television exposure in children after a terrorist incident. Psychiatry Interpers Biolog Processes. 2001;64:202–11.
44. Ray M, Malhi P. Reactions of Indian adolescents to the 9/11 terrorist attacks. Indian J Pediat. 2005;72:217–21.
45. Holmes EA, Creswell C, O'Connor TG. Posttraumatic stress symptoms in London school children following September 11, 2001: an exploratory investigation of peri-traumatic reactions and intrusive imagery. J Behav Ther Exp Psychiatry. 2007;38:474–90.
46. Raccanello D, Burro R, Brondino M, et al. Relevance of terrorism for Italian students not directly exposed to it: the affective impact of the 2015 Paris and the 2016 Brussels attacks. Stress Health. 2018;34:338–43.
47. Pfefferbaum B, Thomas WS, Brandt EN Jr, et al. Media exposure in children one hundred miles from a terrorist bombing. Ann Clin Psychiatry; 15.
48. Phillips D, Prince S, Schiebelhut L. Elementary school children's responses 3 months after the September 11 terrorist attacks: a study in Washington, DC. Am J Orthopsychiatry. 2004;74:509–28.
49. Younis S, Jami H, Riaz F, et al. Adolescent's mental health in context of indirect exposure to terrorism: a qualitative study. J Child Adolesc Trauma. 2025;18:151–65.
50. Otto MW, Henin A, Hirshfeld-Becker DR, et al. Posttraumatic stress disorder symptoms following media exposure to tragic events: impact of 9/11 on children at risk for anxiety disorders. J Anxiety Disord. 2007;21:888–902.
51. Self-Brown SR, Massetti GM, Chen J, et al. Parents' retrospective reports of youth psychological responses to the sniper attacks in the Washington, DC, area. Violence Vict. 2011;26:116–29.
52. Comer JS, Furr JM, Beidas RS, et al. Children and terrorism-related news: training parents in coping and media literacy. J Consult Clin Psychol. 2008;76:568–78.
53. Comer JS, Furr JM, Beidas RS, et al. Media use and children's perceptions of societal threat and personal vulnerability. J Clin Child Adolesc Psychol. 2008;37:622–30.
54. Atwood JD, Donnelly JW. The children's war: their reactions to devastating events. Fam J. 2002;10:11–8.
55. Pfefferbaum B, Pfefferbaum RL, Gurwitch RH, et al. Children's response to terrorism: a critical review of the literature. Curr Psychiatry Rep. 2003;5:95–100.
56. Pfefferbaum B, Sconzo GM, Flynn BW, et al. Case finding and mental health services for children in the aftermath of the Oklahoma City bombing. J Behav Health Serv Res. 2003;30:215–27.
57. Van Overmeire R, Six S, Vesentini L, et al. Questions and emotions of minors after terrorist attacks: a qualitative study using data from a Belgian youth-helpline. Community Ment Health J. 2020;56:280–6.
58. Felix E, Vernberg EM, Pfefferbaum RL, et al. Schools in the shadow of terrorism: psychosocial adjustment and interest in interventions following terror attacks. Psychol Sch. 2010;47:592–605.
59. Pfefferbaum B, Tucker P, Nitiéma P, et al. Inconclusive findings in studies of the link between media coverage of mass trauma and depression in children. Curr Psychiatry Rep. 2022;24:181–93.
60. Robert M, Stene LE, Garfin DR, et al. Media exposure and post-traumatic stress symptoms in the wake of the November 2015 Paris terrorist attacks: a population-based study in France. Front Psychiatry; 12. Epub ahead of print 21 May 2021. https://doi.org/10.3389/fpsyt.2021.509457.

61. Van Overmeire R, Van Keer R, Bilsen J. Impact of terrorist attacks on social relationships. Clin Psychol Psychother. 2021;28:1472–81.
62. Van Overmeire R, Muysewinkel E, Van Keer R-L, et al. Victims of the terrorist attacks in Belgium and professional mental health aid barriers: a qualitative study. Front Psychiatry; 12. Epub ahead of print 2 July 2021. https://doi.org/10.3389/fpsyt.2021.638272.
63. Durodié B, Wainwright D. Terrorism and post-traumatic stress disorder: a historical review. Lancet Psychiatry. 2019;6:61–71.
64. Schlenger WE, Caddell JM, Ebert L, et al. Psychological reactions to terrorist attacks. JAMA. 2002;288:581.
65. Pfefferbaum B, Palka JM, North CS. Associations between news media coverage of the 11 September attacks and depression in employees of New York City area businesses. Behav Sci. 2021;11:29.
66. Ford JD, Adams ML, Dailey WF. Psychological and health problems in a geographically proximate population time-sampled continuously for three months after the September 11th, 2001 terrorist incidents. Anxiety Stress Coping. 2007;20:129–46.
67. Roese NJ, Vohs KD. Hindsight bias. Perspect Psychol Sci. 2012;7:411–26.
68. Kleinman A. The illness narratives: suffering, healing, and the human condition. Basic Books; 1988.
69. Heider F. The psychology of interpersonal relations. Hoboken: Wiley, 1958. Epub ahead of print 1958. https://doi.org/10.1037/10628-000.
70. Kelley HH. The processes of causal attribution. Am Psychol. 1973;28:107–28.
71. Jankowitz S. The 'hierarchy of victims' in Northern Ireland: a framework for critical analysis. Int J Transit Justice. 2018;12:216–36.
72. Paulhus DL. Measurement and control of response bias. In: Measures of personality and social psychological attitudes. Elsevier; 1991. p. 17–59.
73. Bass E, Kaplan-Liss E. A challenging empirical question: what are the effects of media on psychogenic illness during a community crisis? J Community Med Health Educ; 02. Epub ahead of print 2012. https://doi.org/10.4172/jcmhe.1000118.
74. Pfefferbaum B, Weems CF, Scott BG, et al. Research methods in child disaster studies: a review of studies generated by the September 11, 2001, terrorist attacks; the 2004 Indian Ocean Tsunami; and Hurricane Katrina. Child Youth Care Forum. 2013;42:285–337.
75. Van Overmeire R. The association between exposure to terrorist attacks and mental health in Belgium. Thesis, Vrije Universiteit Brussel, 2021.
76. Breslau N, Bohnert KM, Koenen KC. The 9/11 terrorist attack and posttraumatic stress disorder revisited. J Nerv Ment Dis. 2010;198:539–43.
77. Park CL, Aldwin CM, Fenster JR, et al. Pathways to posttraumatic growth versus posttraumatic stress: coping and emotional reactions following the September 11, 2001, terrorist attacks. Am J Orthopsychiatry. 2008;78:300–12.
78. Holman EA, Silver RC, Poulin M, et al. Terrorism, acute stress, and cardiovascular health. Arch Gen Psychiatry. 2008;65:73.
79. Gump BB, Reihman J, Stewart P, et al. Terrorism and cardiovascular responses to acute stress in children. Health Psychol. 2005;24:594–600.
80. Allegra JR. Cardiac events in New Jersey after the September 11, 2001, terrorist attack. J Urban Health. 2005;82:358–63.
81. Remch M, Laskaris Z, Flory J, et al. Post-traumatic stress disorder and cardiovascular diseases. Circ Cardiovasc Qual Outcomes; 11. Epub ahead of print July 2018. https://doi.org/10.1161/CIRCOUTCOMES.117.004572.
82. Goldberg RJ, Spencer F, Lessard D, et al. Occurrence of acute myocardial infarction in Worcester, Massachusetts, before, during, and after the terrorists attacks in New York City and Washington, DC, on 11 September 2001. Am J Cardiol. 2005;95:258–60.
83. Feng J, Lenihanx DJ, Johnson MM, et al. Cardiac sequelae in Brooklyn after the September 11 terrorist attacks. Clin Cardiol. 2006;29:13–7.

84. Strand LB, Mukamal KJ, Halasz J, et al. Short-term public health impact of the July 22, 2011, terrorist attacks in Norway: a nationwide register-based study. Psychosom Med. 2016;78:525–31.
85. Chatignoux E, Gabet A, Moutengou E, et al. The 2015 and 2016 terrorist attacks in France: was there a short-term impact on hospitalizations for cardiovascular disease? Clin Epidemiol. 2018;10:413–9.
86. Eskenazi B, Marks AR, Catalano R, et al. Low birthweight in New York city and upstate New York following the events of September 11th. Hum Reprod. 2007;22:3013–20.
87. El-Sayed A, Hadley C, Galea S. Birth outcomes among Arab Americans in Michigan before and after the terrorist attacks of September 11, 2001. Ethn Dis. 2008;18:348–56.
88. Sherrieb K, Norris FH. Public health consequences of terrorism on maternal–child health in New York City and Madrid. J Urban Health. 2013;90:369–87.
89. Hansen BT, Østergaard SD, Sønderskov KM, et al. Increased incidence rate of trauma- and stressor-related disorders in denmark after the September 11, 2001, terrorist attacks in the United States. Am J Epidemiol. 2016;184:494–500.
90. Hansen BT, Dinesen PT, Østergaard SD. Increased incidence rate of trauma- and stressor-related disorders in Denmark after the Breivik attacks in Norway. Epidemiology. 2017;28:906–9.
91. Franz VA, Glass CR, Arnkoff DB, et al. The impact of the September 11th terrorist attacks on psychiatric patients: a review. Clin Psychol Rev. 2009;29:339–47.
92. Gouraud C, Airagnes G, Kab S, et al. Changes in benzodiazepine use in the French general population after November 2015 terrorist attacks in Paris: an interrupted time series analysis of the national CONSTANCES cohort. BMJ Open. 2021;11:e044891.
93. Karimi A, Bazyar J, Malekyan L, et al. Prevalence of suicidal ideation and suicide attempts after disaster and mass casualty incidents in the world: a systematic review and meta-analysis. Iran J Psychiatry. 2022;17:99–109.
94. Starkman MN. The terrorist attacks of September 11, 2001, as psychological toxin. J Nerv Ment Dis. 2006;194:547–50.
95. Mezuk B, Larkin GL, Prescott MR, et al. The influence of a major disaster on suicide risk in the population. J Trauma Stress. 2009;22:481–8.
96. Claassen CA, Carmody T, Stewart SM, et al. Effect of 11 September 2001 terrorist attacks in the USA on suicide in areas surrounding the crash sites. Br J Psychiatry. 2010;196:359–64.
97. de Lange AW, Neeleman J. The effect of the September 11 terrorist attacks on suicide and deliberate self-harm: a time trend study. Suicide Life Threat Behav. 2004;34:439–47.
98. Salib E. Effect of 11 September 2001 on suicide and homicide in England and Wales. Br J Psychiatry. 2003;183:207–12.
99. Medenwald D. The terror attacks of 9/11 and suicides in Germany. Medicine. 2016;95:e3228.
100. Van Overmeire R, Gidron Y, Six S, et al. Suicide in Flanders, Belgium, after terrorist attacks. Psychol Health Med. 2022;27:1507–13.
101. Vuorio A, Laukkala T, Junttila I, et al. Aircraft-assisted pilot suicides in the general aviation increased for one-year period after 11 September 2001 attack in the United States. Int J Environ Res Public Health. 2018;15:2525.
102. Durkheim E. Suicide. Routledge, 2005. Epub ahead of print 4 August 2005. https://doi.org/10.4324/9780203994320.
103. Na PJ, Bommersbach T, Pietrzak RH, et al. Durkheim's theory of social integration and suicide revisited. J Clin Psychiatry; 84. Epub ahead of print 5 December 2022. https://doi.org/10.4088/JCP.22m14477.
104. Phillips DP. The influence of suggestion on suicide: substantive and theoretical implications of the werther effect. Am Sociol Rev. 1974;39:340.
105. Fink DS, Santaella-Tenorio J, Keyes KM. Increase in suicides the months after the death of Robin Williams in the US. PLoS One. 2018;13:e0191405.
106. Niederkrotenthaler T, Fu K, Yip PSF, et al. Changes in suicide rates following media reports on celebrity suicide: a meta-analysis. J Epidemiol Community Health. 1978;2012(66):1037–42.

107. Von Goethe JW. The sorrows of young werther. Pinguin Classics; 1989.
108. Thompson RR, Holman EA, Silver RC. Worst life events and media exposure to terrorism in a nationally representative U.S. sample. J Trauma Stress. 2020;33:984–93.
109. Huddy L, Feldman S. Americans respond politically to 9/11: understanding the impact of the terrorist attacks and their aftermath. Am Psychol. 2011;66:455–67.
110. Rubin GJ, Brewin CR, Greenberg N, et al. Enduring consequences of terrorism: 7-month follow-up survey of reactions to the bombings in London on 7 July 2005. Br J Psychiatry. 2007;190:350–6.
111. Bove V, Efthyvoulou G, Ghazaryan A, et al. The emotional effect of terrorism. Sci Rep. 2024;14:26525.
112. Healy AF, Aylward AG, Bourne LE, Jr, et al. Terrorism after 9/11: reactions to simulated news reports. Am J Psychol; 122.
113. Ai AL, Cascio T, Santangelo LK, et al. Hope, meaning, and growth following the September 11, 2001, terrorist attacks. J Interpers Violence. 2005;20:523–48.
114. Giner-Sorolla R, Maitner AT. Angry at the unjust, scared of the powerful. Personal Soc Psychol Bull. 2013;39:1069–82.
115. Kim J. The effects of collective anger and fear on policy support in response to terrorist attacks. J Soc Psychol. 2016;156:455–68.
116. Arnoso-Martínez M, Bobowik M, González-Ortega N, et al. News media consumption and support for counter-terrorism measures: the role of hatred and fear. J Soc Psychol. 2025;165:374–89.
117. Goodwin R, Kaniasty K, Sun S, et al. Psychological distress and prejudice following terror attacks in France. J Psychiatr Res. 2017;91:111–5.
118. Laido Z, Till B, Niederkrotenthaler T. Short-term effects of media reports on terrorism that are consistent vs. not consistent with media recommendations on mass shootings: a randomized controlled trial. Suicide Life Threat Behav. 2020;50:948–62.
119. Wild J. Commuters remain stoical in face of terrorist attacks. Nature. 2005;437:13.
120. Rubin GJ, Brewin CR, Greenberg N, et al. Psychological and behavioural reactions to the bombings in London on 7 July 2005: cross sectional survey of a representative sample of Londoners. BMJ. 2005;331:606.
121. Samari; Goleen. Islamophobia and public health in the United States. Am J Public Health. 2016;106:e13.
122. Bulbulia JA, Afzali MU, Yogeeswaran K, et al. Long-term causal effects of far-right terrorism in New Zealand. PNAS Nexus; 2. Epub ahead of print 1 August 2023. https://doi.org/10.1093/pnasnexus/pgad242.
123. Byrne KG, Yogeeswaran K, Dorahy MJ, et al. Author Correction: Psychological impact of far-right terrorism against Muslim minorities on national distress, community, and wellbeing. Sci Rep. 2022;12:2413.
124. Gigerenzer G. Out of the frying pan into the fire: behavioral reactions to terrorist attacks. Risk Anal. 2006;26:347–51.
125. Ormerod P. Why most things fail… And how to avoid it. Faber and Faber; 2005.
126. Handley RV, Salkovskis PM, Scragg P, et al. Clinically significant avoidance of public transport following the London bombings: travel phobia or subthreshold posttraumatic stress disorder? J Anxiety Disord. 2009;23:1170–6.
127. Handley RV, Salkovskis PM, Ehlers A. Treating clinically significant avoidance of public transport following the London bombings? Behav Cogn Psychother. 2009;37:87–93.
128. SCHULDEN J, CHEN J, KRESNOW M, et al. Psychological responses to the sniper attacksWashington DC area, October 2002. Am J Prev Med. 2006;31:324–327.
129. Crum KI, Cornacchio D, Coxe S, et al. Conduct problems among Boston-area youth following the 2013 Marathon bombing: the moderating role of prior violent crime exposure. J Clin Child Adolesc Psychol. 2017;46:343–52.
130. Weiss L. A vulnerable population in a time of crisis: drug users and the attacks on the World Trade Center. J Urban Health. 2002;79:392–403.

131. Factor SH. Drug use frequency among street-recruited heroin and cocaine users in Harlem and the Bronx before and after September 11, 2001. J Urban Health. 2002;79:404–8.
132. Bel S. Nota terroristische aanslagen in België. Brussels; 2017.
133. Hara T. ESTIMATING THE IMMEDIATE EFFECTS OF AN UNPRECEDENTED EVENT OF TERRORISM. Adv Hospit Leisure; 1.
134. Ursano RJ, Fullerton CS, Weisaeth L, et al. Textbook of disaster psychiatry. Cambridge; 2017.
135. Garvey J, Mullins M. Contemporary terrorism: risk perception in the London options market. Risk Anal. 2008;28:151–60.
136. Calderoni ME, Alderman EM, Silver EJ, et al. The mental health impact of 9/11 on inner-city high school students 20 miles north of ground zero. J Adolesc Health. 2006;39:57–65.

# Chapter 5
# Another Side of Trauma: Resilience and Post-traumatic Growth

## 5.1 Introduction

*"I had burning questions. I was mostly wondering why I wasn't more messed up. I was really puzzled, you know. If everybody gets PTSD, why was I doing okay? That was my question, really. Why was I doing okay?"* [1] The question posed by Jed, a survivor of 9/11, who is described in Bonnano's (quite dramatically named) book "The end of trauma," is at the heart of this chapter.

A common critique of disaster research is the focus on mental health problems. Some have raised questions on the cultural focus on mental health issues, since this was not always the case [2, 3]. As Furedi [2] has stated "*Some of the leading figures of American disaster research even concluded that the social impact of disasters was not purely negative and drew attention to studies that indicated that in 'some cases disasters have been beneficial to the victims involved'.*"

This fits the overall idea of the culture of "victimhood," where the concentration of culture is more on those who suffer, and where more things are seen to cause suffering, than on those who are unaffected [4]. Indeed, previous chapters focused on those that develop mental health issues, even though most do not develop mental health issues, and among those that develop post-traumatic stress disorder (PTSD), there can also be post-traumatic growth (PTG) after trauma.

Thus, considering such critique, in this chapter "another side" of terrorism exposure is viewed through the concepts of resilience and post-traumatic growth (PTG). These concepts can be seen as "another side" in the sense that the majority of research focusses on mental health *problems*, while these two concepts imply a view that focuses on either the lack of problems, or even improvement after experiencing an attack.

In this chapter, these concepts will be discussed, starting with definitions and then the research on the concept. The first concept discussed is resilience—though,


R. Van Overmeire, *Terrorism, Mental Health and Aftercare*,
https://doi.org/10.1007/978-3-032-31560-1_5

as will be shown, a large section will be theoretical, namely: the problem of defining resilience.

## 5.2 Resilience

### *5.2.1 Resilience Is a Common Outcome After Terrorism*

Research shows that resilience is a common outcome after terrorism [5]. Bonanno's studies after 9/11 were among the first to show that terrorism does not affect (in terms of long-term mental health issues) a majority of people. In fact, in a landmark study, he and colleagues showed that over 50%—and closer to two thirds—did not develop any or only one PTSD symptom [5, 6]. That is important to expand upon. For example, if a study found 30% of a population having PTSD, that does not necessarily mean the rest of the population has no symptoms of PTSD. In fact, as shown in Chap. 1, some studies employ a so-called partial PTSD screening, where not all requirements for PTSD are met, but the number of issues is still quite high (this type of cutting up findings is especially currant in French terrorism studies). While this method has its uses and limitations, what is interesting here is that Bonanno's studies showed that it is not partial PTSD that is the 70% to the 30% PTSD of the hypothetical study mentioned earlier; what is beyond the 30% PTSD is people having *no* symptoms related to a disorder [6–9].

Studies after 9/11 show that while heavy exposure is related to higher PTSD, there is even resilience here [10]. For example, while people high up in the floors of the World Trade Center had higher PTSD risk than those not in the towers, here too resilience was high [11, 12].

In addition, resilience studies point to the same risk factors for survivors, though show clearer what should be focussed on. For example, socio-economic status is a better indicator for both risk (e.g. lower educated people) as related to resilience (e.g. higher educated). Similarly, social support is related to resilience, while having a chronic disease or mental health issues before the attacks affect it, as will experiencing other stressor events after the attacks [13–16].

In summary, resilience research shows what has been repeated in previous chapters, but from a different angle, namely:

1. A minority of people will develop mental health issues after terrorism.
2. A majority will be resilient after terrorism.

### 5.2.2 *One Concept, Many Interpretations*

So far, this chapter avoided defining resilience, for reasons that will become obvious in this section. In short, defining resilience, while seemingly straightforward (e.g. the name is what it is), it is surprisingly complex. Though attempts have been made to cut out the fat out of the discussion on defining resilience in this section, the following paragraphs should be seen as a snapshot of the discussions on defining it, rather than the final judgement.

Resilience can, in some ways, be seen as the quick recovery or absence of symptoms after trauma. Defining resilience further than this is not easy and will already go against certain conceptualizations. Resilience is not defined in the Diagnostic and Statistical Manual of Mental Disorders (DSM) nor the International Classification of Diseases (ICD), and as such, there is no shared definition. In fact, this is a major obstacle in discussing resilience and it has made the field into a kingdom of separate islands.

For example, while Bonanno et al. [6, 13] (in early studies of Bonanno) sees it as absence of symptoms, in other studies [17] it is measured, theoretically leading to the possibility of someone having both PTSD and being resilient at the same time. In short, resilience has been defined as many different things, whether as a trait, a process, or an outcome [18–20]. All these different meanings have different implications for what the reason for the resilience is.

Thus, the term resilience is used sometimes to indicate something very different, even within terrorism and disaster research, and without actually explaining the meaning of the term, authors often misunderstand each other [18]. For example, some authors differentiate between resistance and resilience [21, 22].. In one study, this is done as follows "*In the first trajectory, termed the resistance trajectory, individuals never develop symptoms of disorder. A second trajectory, termed the resilience trajectory, is characterized by initial symptoms followed by recovery. The resilience trajectory is characterized by improvement to levels that indicate absence of psychological symptoms.*" [22].

Thus, here, resilience does include short term distress. However, this differentiation quickly leads to confusion. In Hobfoll et al.'s [23] conclusion, they state "*[…] Bonanno et al. (2006) found that resistance of Manhattan residents following the World Trade Center attacks, defined by an absence of symptoms assessed at one time point, was not less than 50% for most groups and never fell below one third for even the most exposed groups.*" However, Bonanno et al. [10] never use resistance as term and instead uses resilience as term. In fact, Bonanno et al. [8] has as categories chronic dysfunction, recovery, resilience, and delayed reactions, where recovery is the category that Norris et al. [21] calls resilience.

Thus, what is resistance for one, is resilience for another, and what is a stress response, can still be resilience. This just to give an example of the issues of defining bottom-up (e.g. researchers having no shared framework or definition, and thus define it themselves), instead of top-down (e.g. the DSM or ICD, which, despite their issues, provide a roughly shared definition for all—even though it is seldom follow exactly).

Furthermore, conceptual unclarity across different studies leads to different explanations for what *causes* resilience. For example, one study suggest that six factors are important to facilitate the psychosocial factors underlying resilience: optimism, cognitive flexibility, active coping skills, physical health, social support network, personal moral compass [23]. However, the naming of such factors puts resilience sometimes in danger of becoming self-explanatory: *some people do not develop mental health issues after disaster because they are resilient, and they are resilient because of the factors that they do not have mental health issues after the disasters.* Resilient people are resilient, and their resilience comes from resilience; or in other words, hindsight is 20/20.

This relates to the resilience-paradox: the inability to predict future resilience despite studying resilience [5]. As Bonanno [5] notes, most factors found at one point explaining resilience, do not explain the resilience for future trauma exposure. In other words, what works for an individual to be resilient one day, does not the other day.

There are multiple reasons why resilience research has a bad track record at predicting future resilience.

1. Resilience studies have been mostly cross-sectional studies [5]; meaning that they only have one data point and use that data point to make predictions about the future (as well as the past) resilience of groups. This is also problematic considering that PTSD can have a delayed onset. Meaning that people that appear resilient in one point, might actually have PTSD later on [24]. In fact, one of the critiques on early resilience research had been that resilience does not hold when it keeps being put under pressure, and while all psychosocial resources get exhausted [25, 26].
2. Furthermore, such studies have often relied on single questionaires [5]. The timing of when one measures resilience will therefore matter quite a lot. Such questionnaires sometimes broaden the resilience concept. For example, some include questions on spirituality [5], which seems to indicate that one's spirituality is connected with one's resilience, despite a lack of evidence that spiritual people are more resilient, or vice versa [5].
3. Related to this is what has already been shown earlier in this chapter, namely that resilience has been defined as many different things: it can be a natural ability, something one gets through hardship, et cetera. Naturally, the problem is, is that some of these approaches will be simply untrue. As some authors have pointed out, the idea of resilience being the result of going through hardship seems to lack concrete evidence [7]. While the DSM and ICD clearly define PTSD (and

even then, so many idiosyncratic approaches exist [27]), resilience has no such luck.
4. What works as resilience in one circumstance, has no guarantee to work in another. Meaning, if someone is resilient after a terrorist attack on a shopping mall, they might not be so resilient after an attack on an airplane, which might be due to the personal connection to things, or other circumstances. In fact, during one trauma, someone might have a strong support network, good career, and be happy in life, while after another trauma they might be divorced with no job.
5. Another aspect of it is, is that what people report as stress and no stress might not be related to objective measures. For example, some studies have shown that those who report to have "no stress" sometimes do measure positive for stress based on physical reactions [28]. The other side of it is, is that people who state that they have stress might do so out of a form of social conformity [29]. As such, these are the limits of self-reported questionnaires.

These factors might explain the sometimes large differences between studies. The previously mentioned Hobfoll et al. [22] study shows that the majority of people under continuous terrorist threat are distressed, not resilient, countering the finding of Bonanno et al. [6] that the majority of people after terrorist attacks will be resilient.

However, in recent years, there seems to be more a move towards a common acceptance that indeed, resilience is more common than uncommon [5, 7]. In attempts to come to a shared view, Bonanno and Westphal wrote what they see as the "axioms" of resilience research [7]:

a) Resilience is a common outcome.
b) There are no "key" traits to resilience; as such, resilience is not a type.
c) Resilient outcomes occur through flexible self-regulation.

In the following section, axiom a will be examined for terrorism research.

## 5.3 Post-traumatic Growth

### *5.3.1 Growing After Despair*

While resilience is a form of adaptability, post-traumatic growth is the way one thrives after trauma. This idea is a quite old, philosophical one; namely that out of despair comes insight and truth. The philosopher Soren Kierkegaard describes this, arguably, best in his book "The Sickness unto Death": "*Is despair a merit or a defect? Purely dialectically it is both*" [30]. This is at the essence of this chapter.

Similarly to resilience, many definitions exist of PTG, but PTG is slightly more straightforward to define, as it assumes that someone is affected by trauma. Thus, the question is mainly in what areas a person grows after trauma. As such, the definition of Tedeschi and Calhoun [31] covers the basic principle of resilience: PTG can be defined as the way in which trauma exposure can change one's life in a significant positive way [31].

### 5.3.2 Growth After Terrorism

To illustrate PTG, it is useful to quote survivors of the Christchurch Mosque attacks in New-Zealand:

> "Re-prioritising, re-thinking what I want to do, and what my life will involve … I've reduced a lot of my workload … And just kind of chosen to do what I love".
>
> "That I noted that there's a difference in me and I'm cherishing every … I read a book, I play some things like games, go for a walk … I start actually running this morning".
>
> "A lot more closeness with my Dad, my sister, and family overseas that were not together. Definitely a sense of closeness, but also within the Muslim community" [32].

Thus, while resilience is the status-quo after disaster, post-traumatic growth is a positive change after disaster, that can include a greater appreciation for life, existentialistic concern for human life and vulnerability, as well as a deeper feeling of religiousness or spirituality [32–35]. Like resilience, it is not uncommon. In fact, after the previously mentioned Christchurch attacks around half of those with PTSD had PTG [36].

However, that observation also leads to what is another major observation about PTG: while it is, like PTSD, linked to exposure to trauma, it is also linked to PTSD; in other words, PTG and PTSD is associated with PTSD [37–43], and with anger [44]. Thus, it is not surprising that PTG does not suppress PTSD and that resilience and PTG are negatively associated: the less resilience, the more change for PTG [40]. Thus, studies show that severe distress seems to be necessary for PTG [45]. This association between PTSD and PTG is noticed in studies on terrorist attacks, whether the Oslo bombing, Spain, Israel or Oklahoma [33, 42, 45, 46]. For example, among the majority of survivors of the Oslo attacks, there was also evidence of post-traumatic growth, indicating a new appreciation of parts of life and others [47].

However, there is not enough evidence concerning the association in the long-term [45]. One study, 18.5 years after the Oklahoma City Bombing, showed that heavily exposed survivors with PTSD still reported PTG [33], while 15 years after 9/11, PTG was found to be present among those with high exposure, who had high social support, but also, who had high PTSD initially [48], indicating that PTSD can fade with time, and leave behind PTG.

The way this PTG occurs, can be different. For example, after attacks in Spain, there was more appreciation of life, less spiritual change and less relating to others compared to for example the findings of the Oklahoma City Bombing study [45]. It seems to indicate that cultural factors matter in how the PTG is experienced. For example, in more collective oriented societies (e.g. Japan), social bonds and collective meaning making of disasters seem to help in creating post-traumatic growth [49]. In addition, there is some evidence that PTG is also related to attribution, which means that it matters for people whether a disaster was man-made or a natural disaster [50].

PTG might at first sight seem as a positive aspect, as Furedi [2] seems to indicate in the quote mentioned at the beginning of this chapter, but clearly it goes hand in hand with PTSD. Even more so, studies among veterans show that this PTG can also have negative ramifications, such as an increased loneliness due to feeling less understood by other [51].

### *5.3.3 The Janus Face of Growth*

How can be PTG be a positive growth and at the same time has such clear links with PTSD? It might be that PTG is, partly, a matter of illusion. It is important to first recollect that most of the studies cited in this book are self-reported, and also the ones on PTG in general, are self-reported studies, meaning that survivors of trauma answer themselves whether they have grown or not grown, yet people with PTSD after traumatic experiences might deny certain aspects of what they are experiencing [52, 53]. That is in fact something that has been observed in interviews with terrorism survivors, who ignored mental health issues to uphold social roles or to not appear weak, among other reasons [54].

As such, Maercker and Zoellner [52] have called it a "Janus face model," named after the Roman god Janus, who had two faces: one looking to the past, and one looking for the future. Similarly, the Janus face model indicates that PTG can be both a transcending experiencing (forward looking), and also a self-deceiving experience (due to the PTSD; which is the part that is looking at the past, as it can consist of memory related issues, such as flashbacks, triggers due to the trauma, nightmares, etc) [52]. In fact, several studies indeed seem to show that survivors of traumatic experiences deceive themselves that the traumatic experience led to growth for them as a way of coping with the events [55, 56].

## 5.4 Conclusions

This chapter provided a brief snapshot of the discussions in resilience, as well as some results of the field, while also providing insights into post-traumatic growth. However, what can be concluded from another view of terrorism research?

First, that most people will move on from exposure to terrorism. While certainly they will never forget the trauma, it will also not define their mental health. For those that do develop severe distress, it can also be, surprisingly perhaps, a transformative experience.

Secondly, resilience studies show also the need to look broader. Trauma exposure is often used as catch-all to explaining mental health symptoms, despite that trauma exposure is in itself not uncommon [57], and that most people who experience symptoms after trauma, already had some form of mental health issues *before* the trauma [58].

From a policy perspective, the conclusion is that early interventions after terrorism should focus more on risk groups than on whole populations: people with low socio-economic status, with a chronic illness, those who suffer income loss due to the attacks… [13] From a cost-efficiency, it seems more opportune that focussed interventions are employed, considering that most people will in fact not develop any issues. Such early interventions should also not be psychological in nature, but provide social support [59]. In fact, as a later chapter will shows, social support is the greatest buffer against the development of PTSD [60]. As another later chapter will show, organizing such interventions is not easy, and requires quite a lot of planning ahead, but does save burden for a significant number of people overall.

Adding to this policy perspective, it is important to note that terms such as resilience and PTG do not mean that survivors do not need help. Yes, aid could be more targeted; yes, society is quite resilient, but resilience is not universal; it is a majority, but not everyone. The danger of resilience approaches is that, as Jore noted about resilience in terrorism research in general, it might become an ideological goal [61]. Indeed, there are studies showing that survivors of terrorism have difficulty to receive any reimbursement from the government, unless they have physical wounds, due to the inability to prove their mental health issues [54]. A resilience view of survivors might lead societies back towards the view that only physical wounds have meaning, and that one's mental health is, at most, secondary.

That does not mean that governments should promote victimhood. Anything but! In fact, perhaps it would be useful to promote resilience to the general public after attacks [3]. Clearly, societies are strong, but it remains important to also provide the necessary aid to those survivors of an attack that was not aimed against them personally but aimed against their state.

Similarly, to resilience, post-traumatic growth should not be romanticised. It is evidence of people's ability to adjust, and strive, yes, but PTG is also linked with anger issues, loneliness, and other aspects typical for people with PTSD. PTG is the silver-lining, and perhaps even useful to keep in mind when providing therapy to people with PTSD: there is possibility to come out of PTSD with a new worldview, and more appreciation for life.

## References

1. Bonanno GA. The end of trauma. New York: Basic Books; 2021.
2. Furedi F. The changing meaning of disaster. Area. 2007;39:482–9.
3. Durodié B, Wainwright D. Terrorism and post-traumatic stress disorder: a historical review. Lancet Psychiatry. 2019;6:61–71.
4. Campbell B, Manning J. The rise of victimhood culture. Cham: Springer International, 2018. Epub ahead of print 2018. https://doi.org/10.1007/978-3-319-70329-9.
5. Bonanno GA. The resilience paradox. Eur J Psychotraumatol; 12. Epub ahead of print 30 January 2021. https://doi.org/10.1080/20008198.2021.1942642.

6. Bonanno GA. Loss, trauma, and human resilience: have we underestimated the human capacity to thrive after extremely aversive events? Am Psychol. 2004;59:20–8.
7. Bonanno GA, Westphal M. The three axioms of resilience. J Trauma Stress. 2024;37:717–23.
8. Bonanno GA, Mancini AD. The human capacity to thrive in the face of potential trauma. Pediatrics. 2008;121:369–75.
9. Bonanno GA, Westphal M, Mancini AD. Resilience to loss and potential trauma. Annu Rev Clin Psychol. 2011;7:511–35.
10. Bonanno GA, Galea S, Bucciarelli A, et al. Psychological resilience after disaster. Psychol Sci. 2006;17:181–6.
11. DiGrande L, Neria Y, Brackbill RM, et al. Long-term posttraumatic stress symptoms among 3,271 civilian survivors of the September 11, 2001, terrorist attacks on the World Trade Center. Am J Epidemiol. 2011;173:271–81.
12. Gargano LM, Nguyen A, DiGrande L, et al. Mental health status of World Trade Center tower survivors compared to other survivors a decade after the September 11, 2001 terrorist attacks. Am J Ind Med. 2016;59:742–51.
13. Bonanno GA, Galea S, Bucciarelli A, et al. What predicts psychological resilience after disaster? The role of demographics, resources, and life stress. J Consult Clin Psychol. 2007;75:671–82.
14. Butler LD, Koopman C, Azarow J, et al. Psychosocial predictors of resilience after the September 11, 2001 terrorist attacks. J Nerv Ment Dis. 2009;197:266–73.
15. Butler LD, Morland LA, Leskin GA. Psychological resilience in the face of terrorism. In: Psychology of terrorism. Oxford University Press; 2006. p. 400–17.
16. Mao W, Agyapong VIO. The role of social determinants in mental health and resilience after disasters: implications for public health policy and practice. Front Public Health; 9. Epub ahead of print 19 May 2021. https://doi.org/10.3389/fpubh.2021.658528.
17. Yılmazer E. Psychological distress, resilience, and well-being among survivors of the 2023 Kahramanmaraş earthquakes: a multi-site cross-sectional study. Front Psychol; 16. Epub ahead of print 10 December 2025. https://doi.org/10.3389/fpsyg.2025.1730083.
18. Vella S-L, Pai N. A theoretical review of psychological resilience: defining resilience and resilience research over the decades. Archiv Med Health Sci. 2019;7:233.
19. Windle G. What is resilience? A review and concept analysis. Rev Clin Gerontol. 2011;21:152–69.
20. Fletcher D, Sarkar M. Psychological resilience. Eur Psychol. 2013;18:12–23.
21. Norris FH, Tracy M, Galea S. Looking for resilience: understanding the longitudinal trajectories of responses to stress. Soc Sci Med. 2009;68:2190–8.
22. Hobfoll SE, Palmieri PA, Johnson RJ, et al. Trajectories of resilience, resistance, and distress during ongoing terrorism: the case of Jews and Arabs in Israel. J Consult Clin Psychol. 2009;77:138–48.
23. Iacoviello BM, Charney DS. Psychosocial facets of resilience: implications for preventing posttrauma psychopathology, treating trauma survivors, and enhancing community resilience. Eur J Psychotraumatol; 5. Epub ahead of print 1 December 2014. https://doi.org/10.3402/ejpt.v5.23970.
24. Fischer IC, Pietrzak RH, Maercker A, et al. Post-traumatic stress disorder: rethinking diagnosis. Lancet Psychiatry. 2023;10:741–2.
25. Kelley TM. Natural resilience and innate mental health. Am Psychol. 2005;60:265.
26. Roisman GI. Conceptual clarifications in the study of resilience. Am Psychol. 2005;60:264–5.
27. Muysewinkel E, Stene LE, Van Deynse H, et al. Post-what stress? A review of methods of research on posttraumatic stress during COVID-19. J Anxiety Disord. 2024;102:102829.
28. Roth M, Herzberg PY. The resilient personality prototype. J Individ Differ. 2017;38:1–11.
29. Pfefferbaum B, Seale TW, Mcdonald NB, et al. Posttraumatic stress two years after the Oklahoma City bombing in youths geographically distant from the explosion. Psychiatry. 2000;63:358–70.
30. Kierkegaard S. The sickness unto death. London: Pinguin books; 2004.

31. Tedeschi R, Calhoun L. Trauma and transformation: growing in the aftermath of suffering. Sage Publications; 2012.
32. Dean S, Eggleston K, Ali F, et al. 'I can feel sad about it and I can worry, but inside I know everything happens for a reason': personal experiences in the aftermath of the March 15 Christchurch mosque attacks. BJPsych Open. 2024;10:e176.
33. Tucker P, Pfefferbaum B, Nitiéma P, et al. Intensely exposed Oklahoma City terrorism survivors. J Nerv Ment Dis. 2016;204:203–9.
34. Turner B, Raitt J, Lee MH, et al. Perspectives of survivors of the Oklahoma City bombing with and without PTSD 17 months postdisaster: a qualitative study. J Relig Spiritual Soc Work Soc Thought. 2022;41:308–24.
35. Hong BA, Pollio DE, Pollio EW, et al. Religious and spiritual aspects of disaster experience among survivors of the 9/11 attacks on New York City's World Trade Center. J Relig Health. 2019;58:1619–30.
36. Beaglehole B, Boden JM, Porter R, et al. Post-traumatic growth and religious coping in Muslims exposed to the March 15 terror attacks in New Zealand: a cross-sectional study. Aust N Z J Psychiatry. 2025;59:1019–26.
37. Zalta AK, Gerhart J, Hall BJ, et al. Self-reported posttraumatic growth predicts greater subsequent posttraumatic stress amidst war and terrorism. Anxiety Stress Coping. 2017;30:176–87.
38. Liu A-N, Wang L-L, Li H-P, et al. Correlation between posttraumatic growth and posttraumatic stress disorder symptoms based on pearson correlation coefficient. J Nerv Ment Dis. 2017;205:380–9.
39. Levine SZ, Laufer A, Stein E, et al. Examining the relationship between resilience and posttraumatic growth. J Trauma Stress. 2009;22:282–6.
40. Levine SZ, Laufer A, Hamama-Raz Y, et al. Posttraumatic growth in adolescence: examining its components and relationship with PTSD. J Trauma Stress. 2008;21:492–6.
41. Shechory Bitton M, Laufer A. PTSD and PTG among Israeli mothers: opposite facets of exposure to terrorism. Stress Health. 2017;33:676–83.
42. Blix I, Hansen MB, Birkeland MS, et al. Posttraumatic growth, posttraumatic stress and psychological adjustment in the aftermath of the 2011 Oslo bombing attack. Health Qual Life Outcomes. 2013;11:160.
43. Hall BJ, Hobfoll SE, Canetti D, et al. Exploring the association between posttraumatic growth and PTSD. J Nerv Ment Dis. 2010;198:180–6.
44. Park CL, Aldwin CM, Fenster JR, et al. Pathways to posttraumatic growth versus posttraumatic stress: coping and emotional reactions following the September 11, 2001, terrorist attacks. Am J Orthopsychiatry. 2008;78:300–12.
45. Fausor R, Sanz J, Navarro-McCarthy A, et al. Long-term posttraumatic growth in victims of terrorism in Spain. Front Psychol. 2022;13:847099.
46. Laufer A. Posttraumatic growth and well-being among body handlers: the role of resilience, coping strategies, and belief in a just world. Mil Psychol. 2025:1–11.
47. Glad KA, Czajkowski NO, Dyb G, et al. Does event centrality mediate the effect of peritraumatic reactions on post-traumatic growth in survivors of a terrorist attack? Eur J Psychotraumatol. 2020;11:1766276.
48. Pollari CD, Brite J, Brackbill RM, et al. World Trade Center exposure and posttraumatic growth: assessing positive psychological change 15 years after 9/11. Int J Environ Res Public Health. 2020;18:104.
49. Brooks M, O'Brien RO, Livanou M, et al. Collective violence, strengths, and perceived posttraumatic growth: a scoping review. Trauma Violence Abuse. 2025;26:342–55.
50. Palgi Y, Dicker-Oren SD, Greene T. Evaluating a community fire as human-made vs. natural disaster moderates the relationship between peritraumatic distress and both PTSD symptoms and posttraumatic growth. Anxiety Stress Coping. 2020;33:569–80.
51. Stein JY, Levin Y, Bachem R, et al. Growing apart: a longitudinal assessment of the relation between post-traumatic growth and loneliness among combat veterans. Front Psychol; 9. Epub ahead of print 7 June 2018. https://doi.org/10.3389/fpsyg.2018.00893.

52. Maercker A, Zoellner T. The Janus face of self-perceived growth: toward a two-component model of posttraumatic growth. Psychol Inq; 15.
53. Zoellner T, Maercker A. Posttraumatic growth in clinical psychology — A critical review and introduction of a two component model. Clin Psychol Rev. 2006;26:626–53.
54. Van Overmeire R, Muysewinkel E, Van Keer R-L, et al. Victims of the terrorist attacks in Belgium and professional mental health aid barriers: a qualitative study Front Psychiatry; 12. Epub ahead of print 2 July 2021. https://doi.org/10.3389/fpsyt.2021.638272.
55. McFarland C, Alvaro C. The impact of motivation on temporal comparisons: coping with traumatic events by perceiving personal growth. J Pers Soc Psychol. 2000;79:327–43.
56. Frazier P, Tennen H, Gavian M, et al. Does self-reported posttraumatic growth reflect genuine positive change? Psychol Sci. 2009;20:912–9.
57. Kessler RC, Aguilar-Gaxiola S, Alonso J, et al. Trauma and PTSD in the WHO World mental health surveys. Eur J Psychotraumatol; 8. Epub ahead of print 27 October 2017. https://doi.org/10.1080/20008198.2017.1353383.
58. van der Velden PG, Contino C, Das M, et al. To what extent do post-traumatic mental health and other problems reflect pre-existing problems? Findings from the prospective comparative population-based VICTIMS-study. Int J Soc Psychiatry. 2023;69:841–52.
59. Shalev AY. Further lessons from 9/11: does stress equal trauma? Psychiatry Interpers Biol Process. 2004;67:174–7.
60. Wang Y, Chung MC, Wang N, et al. Social support and posttraumatic stress disorder: a meta-analysis of longitudinal studies. Clin Psychol Rev. 2021;85:101998.
61. Jore SH. Is resilience a favourable concept in terrorism research? The multifaceted discourses of resilience in the academic literature. Crit Stud Terror. 2020;13:337–57.

# Chapter 6
# Crossing Lines: Lessons to Learn from Studies on Disasters, Political Violence, and War

## 6.1 Introduction

The study of mental health after terrorism is often taken together with other studies of the mental health consequences of mass violence, whether political violence or war [1]. This is not illogical. Terrorism and war often go hand in hand, and in fact, terrorism can even lead to situation that are seemingly close to war [2]. For example, ISIS is seen as a terrorist organization in Europe due to their attacks in Paris and Brussels, among others, but in the Levant, ISIS was a military organization that was defeated in a military sense.

Terrorism studies are also often taken together with other forms of disaster, such as natural disasters or technological disasters. In fact, lessons from terrorism have even been applied to the study of the mental health consequences of corona pandemic [3].

In addition, this chapter also serves as counterpart to the tunnel vision that might be experienced towards terrorism. It is no doubt the paradox of any academic book: it should be hyper focused on its subject, while at the same time avoiding tunnel vision. However, it is important to also view populations where terrorism is one of the many trauma exposures, or even a common exposure. For example, in Pakistan, while 34% of the population has post-traumatic stress disorder (PTSD), the most prevalent trauma was domestic violence, followed by terrorism exposure [4]. As other studies have mentioned, focus on single trauma exposure can lead to attributing too much to that single trauma [5].

Finally, lessons can be learned from other areas. Considering the many similarities, there are also ideas and concepts that can be borrowed from other fields.

While it is difficult to learn much with regard to mental health aid interventions, as the resources are completely different across the world and across conflicts, war and other mass violence teach lessons about what is associated with, or causes, mental health problems after disasters or mass violence [2].



R. Van Overmeire, *Terrorism, Mental Health and Aftercare*,
https://doi.org/10.1007/978-3-032-31560-1_6

This chapter will provide both general observations on disasters as case studies, since sometimes a case study is used to showcase historical precedents, or insights that are important, that a general observation on, for example, natural disasters would not provide.

## 6.2 Natural Disasters

Natural disasters have the clearest overlap with terrorism, though there are also differences that highlight the way terrorism has the impact it has.

First, the similarities. Natural disasters can cause high PTSD rates. Reviews summarize that floods have caused around 29.48% PTSD in populations [6], while this is 16.37% for earthquakes [7]. Similarly, these rates tend to go down with time, leaving a minority that has long-term PTSD [8], with some of those with PTSD having post-traumatic growth [9, 10]. Like terrorism as well, the mental health aid usage after the attacks is linked not with PTSD, but with the exposure one has to the disaster: the higher the exposure, the more mental health aid someone will try and seek out [11].

Other more niche observations in terrorism research also hold up for natural disasters. For example, that the stress pregnant women experience due to a natural disaster is bad for their unborn child [12], or that prior trauma is a risk factor, as well as certain socio-demographic factors [13]. This is only normal, considering that stress does not differentiate on the type of disaster. Similarly, there is unclarity on the increased risk of suicide, adding further evidence to the context (e.g. culture) of suicidal behaviour [14].

There are clear differences between terrorism and natural disasters, however.

First, natural disasters come in many different forms, of course, but they often involve wider scale property damage [15, 16]. In the case of fires, in addition to the property damage and economic damage, the fine particles released can be more harmful than any other fine particles [16]. This "environmental" damage in itself is, however, interesting, since this is an area that is often neglected in terrorism research. For example, attacks on old buildings that might contain asbestos (which is quite common in Europe), or simply other circumstantial events. Only studies on 9/11 have shown such insights.

A major conceptual difference with terrorism is that while terrorism will try and attack well-known and populated areas, a natural disaster will, generally, mostly affect people with a low socio-economic status [17]. As Hartman and Squires stated: there is no such thing as a natural disaster [18]. Thus, an important lesson of natural disasters is actually the importance of "attribution" [19]. In other words, it matters whether someone views something as a natural occurrence, or a man-made disaster. It is here that a major difference between terrorism and natural disasters becomes obvious: while natural disasters can be viewed as acts of God, or bad luck, but terrorism, despite the possibility of attributing it as well to acts of God or bad luck, will more often affect one's believe in a just world, create the feeling that world is random, and teach survivors, to quote Fausto Maijstral in Pynchon's novel V, "*Life's single lesson,*" namely "*that there is more accident to [life] than a man can ever admit to in a lifetime and stay sane.*" [20–22].

**The Buffalo Creek Flood**

The Buffalo Creek in West-Virginia ended at a large dam, and in its shadow lay around 16 coal mining towns. On the 26th of February 1972, the dam broke. A raging flood of water swept over the towns, killing hundred, injuring thousands. Kai Erikson studied the survivors afterwards in his landmark studies. He observed that the survivors felt like outcasts of normal life: social ties had been broken in the aftermath, friendships and marriages were lost, and even the ability to connect with others was lost [23]. Trauma, he found, had a social dimension [24].

Yet, while the survivors were excluded from their previous life, they found understanding with those who had experienced it with them. This was not the "post-traumatic growth" mentioned in psychological studies; instead, it was a social renewal. Erikson quotes a Holocaust survivor to explain the patterns he found as well in the survivors of his studies: one Holocaust survivor explained on why she married a fellow Holocaust survivor whom she did not really love:

> He knew who I was – he was the only who knew… And I knew who he was. [24, 25]

Survivors of trauma know each other in ways even the closest friends never will, which can be called "collective trauma" [23, 24]. This collective trauma is the damage trauma does to the social fabric of a community [23]. In fact, while survivors sought comfort with each other, they started viewing others differently, and in fact started viewing humanity as inhuman, and the world as unjust [24].

Here the findings of the chapter on post-traumatic growth can be repeated, but in a different way. As mentioned, some people who experience post-traumatic growth also experienced negative effects, such as loneliness and a feeling that others did not understand them anymore [26]. The survivors of Buffalo Creek certainly changed, grew even, but at the same time, their connection with the world seemed to have been broken [24]. This relates to an important lesson that terrorism studies have not yet incorporated yet, due to an overwhelming psychological focus: to help people in the aftermath of disaster, it is important to also focus on healing the community [27].

**The Corona Pandemic and Research**

During the corona pandemic, an enormous number of studies were being published on PTSD of people worldwide. It is also a period in which very few studies actually properly measured PTSD. In fact, a review showed that roughly 10% of the studies actually measured PTSD with no trauma indicator (thus, many studies could have looked at common stress) [28]. Which is why many COVID-19 studies show PTSD percentages that sometimes go above 90% of the population.

A lesson to be drawn from these generally poorly executed lessons is that preparations are needed for large-scale public health surveys, to have decent measures. After all, if studies show that 60% of students have PTSD, what is public health policy supposed to do?

## 6.3 Technological Disasters

**Train Disasters**

Technological disasters are at the one hand the most *recent* type of disaster to exist on the world (e.g. industrial disasters could not happen in the fifth century, while natural and man-made disasters certainly could), and yet on the other hand, also (arguably) the first studied disasters from a psychological perspective.

During the mid-nineteenth century, the train was quickly becoming a popular form of public transport across Europe, yet, this also came with many accidents. A famous example was that of the American railroader Casey Jones, who seeing a train ahead with which his train would collide, stayed on his train to brake as to minimize the impact. Casey Jones was immortalized in songs such as "The Ballad of Casey Jones" (or more modern, "Casey Jones," by The Grateful Dead, where the accident happened because he was under the influence of cocaine), and so too are the stories remembered of the many people affected after such collisions or train crashes.

For example, the British writer Charles Dickens, who had experienced the Staplehurst railroad catastrophe in 1865, stated:

> I am curiously weak…I begin to feel it more in my head… I turn faint and sick…yesterday I felt more shaken than I have since the accident. I cannot bear railway travelling yet [29].

Following these many train disasters, more and more passengers, despite not being wounded, experienced severe changes in their emotional reactions. They started suing railway companies, demanding reimbursements for their emotional damage. The lawsuits attracted, for one of the first times, great public attention for scientific theories, which tried to explain the mysterious ailments, and tried to verify if these people were malingers or had actual non-visible wounds that affected their functioning [30]. Scientific journals that are now among the most reputable in the world would follow these trials, commenting on the theories and the cases [31].

Doctors of the day tried to provide diagnoses for the emotional reactions. One doctor John Eric Erichsen called it "railway spine" [30–32], based on the idea that the emotional reactions were caused by micro lesions in the back. This was not so surprising, since severe fear reactions were mainly seen to be a physical force, not a mental or psychological force. Therefore, if this fear had such long-lasting consequences, there had to either some form of organic explanation, or some damage to the "nervous apparatus" [30].

What can be learned from these historical precedents, is the search for the "truth" of someone's experiences, even when they are hidden. Furthermore, another lesson to learn from this is that knowledge about post-traumatic reactions (in this, not referring to the diagnosis, but literally to mental health reactions after a traumatic experience) tend to get lost in time, and forgotten. What is true for one group, tends to need to be proven again for another group. That is also the experience of terrorism survivors, who, despite having survived terrorism, often need to prove that they in fact can develop mental health issues because of exposure to the terrorist attacks [33].

**The Bhopal Disaster**

One of the largest disasters ever was in fact a technological disaster, namely the Bhopal disaster.

The Union Carbide India Limited factory at Bhopal, India, developed pesticides. Negligence, poor management, and other factors had caused small gas leaks, and Rajkumar Keswani, a journalist, warned policy makers repeatedly for a possible impending disaster, stating, while referring to a leak in another factory, that when such a leak would occur in Bhopal, "*there will not even be a solitary witness to testify to what took place*" [34].

Methyl-iso-cyanate (MIC) was one of the products being used in the factory for the production of pesticides. After a chemical reaction with water, 40 tons of MIC leaked out in the night of the 3rd of December, 1984 [35]. Around 2000 people died the night itself, which is 1% of those directly exposed. In the following years, thousands more died, with some estimates running up to 25,000, with tens of thousands being injured [36]. It is the largest man-made disaster to have ever occurred, with more victims than 9/11 and Chernobyl.

In the aftermath, there were severe unmet mental health needs of those exposed. Mental health teams were unavailable for 8 weeks, due to a lack of professionals near the scene of the attack. Even up to 30 years later, survivors could experience anxiety, PTSD, and other mental health issues [36].

There were several issues with the mental health aid that are important to note. First, many doctors only provided treatment for physical symptoms and thought the emotional responses of survivors was solely due to get treatment for their physical health [36]. Secondly, the poor coordination of voluntary services resulted in mistrust. Third, the needs of the people of Bhopal would have been met if the focus had been community based, and not individual and clinically based. Not focusing on the community in the aftermath of disaster, leads to the community falling apart [36]. So, while the survivors of the Buffalo Creek flood had each other, sharing their collective trauma [24], the risk exists that the community falls apart (e.g. through migration to other cities), limiting the social support the community can provide [36].

These too are lessons that are important in any public health psychosocial care response after terrorism, and the focus on community is present in Chap. 9.

## 6.4 Political Violence

Political violence (e.g. violent protests) and state violence (e.g. terrorism against the population by the government) both can be related to mental health problems. For example, school children living nearby the Tahrir square in Egypt, experienced symptoms akin to PTSD [37], while around 8% of protesters of the Occupy Central/

Umbrella movement experienced moderate depression [38]. What seems to be protective is having a high socio-economic status, as well as high social support [38]. Such social unrest also seems to affect sleep, and causes distress among all age ranges [39, 40]. Similarly, protests in Kazakhstan that turned into violence show that such events can be linked to distress and slightly higher mental health issues in the population and those exposed to them [41].

Interestingly, even when protests are nonviolent, they also are associated with distress, increasing the chance of depression with 7% even among people not part of the protest, though a few studies also show that being part of a protest can also be beneficial, due to the community spirit [42]. However, overall, it seems protests do cause some form of mental distress in the short term. The feeling togetherness can serve as barrier against the distress [43]. Additionally, that togetherness can arise due to the shared moral injury of protestors [43].

Moral injury is a concept that is not often used in terrorism studies, which is unfortunate. While not having any definite definition, moral injury is the wound that people might feel due to a sense of injustice in a traumatic situation [44]. For example, rescue workers often have to make on-the-spot calls when intervening in the aftermath of terrorism [45], while survivors might feel a sense of injustice due to how their government is treating them [46], yet in terrorism studies, it is not named as such, despite that this moral injury might be applied to the social support bonds created in the aftermath of terrorism (see Chap. 7) as well as predicting PTSD [44]. The few studies after terrorism that have studied this indeed show the importance of moral injury in explaining mental health issues [47].

## 6.5 State Terror

While terrorism can be seen as an attack on the state, state terror is an attack by the state on the people. There is no research on this, which might be because state terror often goes hand in hand with censorship. Additionally, when being oppressed, mental health-studies do not add to addressing that oppression directly. State terror is also not the same as a country in civil war, or at war with another country, which will be discussed later.

As one example of state terror, Chile under Pinochet had been chosen, though there are many other state terror examples, such as the Holocaust.

**Growth After State Terror Under Pinochet in Chile**

On 11 September 1973, a coup d'état took place: the Chilean army, navy, and air force took control of the country. Sitting President Salvador Allende, supposedly, committed suicide with a gun given to him, supposedly again, by Fidel Castro. Somewhat by chance, General Augusto Pinoceht eventually took over, and while originally a rotating leadership was meant to be implemented, the General did not follow that line in the end and intimated the other members that led to coup to accepting this new reality [48].

Pinochet started a dictatorship that focussed on removing any opposition. Within the first 10 days, many leftists were rounded up in sport stadiums and tortured or killed, while afterwards kill squads went from city to city in what has been known as the "Caravan of Death" [49]. Among the thousands of victims of the regime were the folk singer Victor Jara, or (allegedly, once again) the Nobel prize winning poet Pablo Neruda, and thousands were imprisoned and tortured, while the population was constantly monitored by Pinochet's national intelligence agency, DINA. Pinochet's reign ended 17 years later, in 1990 [48].

Those that lived through and survived the state terror, sometimes developed PTSD and other mental health issues [50–55]. Not surprisingly, even in the post-dictatorship time, there is very low institutional trust in Chile, as well as low trust in the economic model [54, 55]. In addition, social relationships were severely damaged throughout society: anyone could betray someone, and everyone could cast suspicion on someone [50].

However, there is also a lot of resilience, and post-traumatic growth [53, 56]. In fact, post-traumatic growth was quite common among survivors of the state terror [50, 53]. Survivors created new meaning in life, and were able to positively appraise the traumatic events [53], and while growth does not mean forgiveness [53], as Cárdenas et al. [50] state "*violence can have a paradoxical effect, as it aims to harm others while opening the door to the discovery of unknown strengths in survivors*".

Such studies showcase several aspects understudied, but important, for terrorism studies. First, institutional trust, and its role in mental health. Very few studies [57] have looked at the role of institutional trust after terrorist attacks, despite that this too is very much related to the state—namely, an attack on the state that affects innocent civilians. Second, the role of post-traumatic growth is shown in these studies, but also that post-traumatic growth is nuanced. It is linked with PTSD, and it does not mean that someone will forgive perpetrators. This last aspect is often not studied in such studies after terrorism.

## 6.6 Being in a War Zone

Whether displaced due to the Sudanese war, or Syrian refugees, all those affected by war had much higher risks for PTSD, depression or anxiety [58]. In some cases, even up to ten times more than the average person [59, 60]. Being in an active war zone is associated with very high PTSD rates, due to many factors related to being in a war zone, whether it is being nearby shooting or being shot at, torture, sexual assault, having no shelter, or many other factors related to the deterioration of one's environment [61].

Experiencing shooting and combat is associated with high PTSD rates. For example, almost 30% of women living in war struck Afghanistan in 2006 had PTSD, which was especially high among those who had directly experienced events involving shootings and combat [62]. Similarly, almost 40% of the general population in South Sudan seemed to suffer from PTSD, even after the signing of the peace treaty and creation of South Sudan [63, 64], which is similar to Ukraine, where almost half suffered from depression and other issues during the Russian invasion of Ukraine [65, 66]. In Ethiopia, almost half of internally displaced people exhibited PTSD, and an eight showing suicidal behaviour, with risk factors including seeing a loved one being killed or being threated, but also having low social support [67, 68]. This low social support can be especially low in women. One study on war-traumatized women in Bosnia and Herzegovina had low support, especially from friends, which increased the risk of developing PTSD [69]. However, family is very important in healing in the post conflict period [70, 71]. In fact, the loss of such social resources during war predicts PTSD [72].

That war zones cause these mental health issues is also evident from studies. Studies in Nepal, before and after the political violence, showed that especially conflict exposure sometimes doubled the mental health issues in the population [73]. Furthermore, these studies showcase that during the conflict, almost half of people displaced due to the violence had PTSD, but that *after* the violence, this lowered to roughly 10% [74, 75]. Important to note that in other studies, this lowering depends on the duration of the displacement [76].

It seems that displacement during war has such a huge mental health impact is due to several factors, such as the need for financial aid, malnutrition, lack of treatment of physical injuries, but also the need for food and shelter for children, and other reasons that are caused because of war [61, 77–79]. That the worry for loved ones causes more mental health issues is also evident from studies during the first months of conflict in Khartoum, where marriage was associated with more mental health issues, possibly because of the continuous stress of having loved ones in danger [80]. In addition, displacement also causes non-violent sources to become larger mortality risks, and this especially for women and children [78].

In addition, war seldom comes alone as disaster. In Myanmar, war was combined with the ongoing COVID-19 pandemic, as well as economic collapse. Across the population of the country, 8.1% had PTSD and roughly 14% depression [81]. It also follows from such a collapse that finding mental health aid is not easy. However, even in post-war countries, stigma still is the biggest limitation in finding mental health aid [82].

Also important to note is that the sense of justice after war (e.g. persecuting war criminals) does not actually lead to less PTSD. In fact, sense of justice is completely separate from PTSD [83]. Then again, PTSD and depression are coupled with the wish to how conflict ends. The more PTSD or depression one has, the more in favour of ending conflict through means of violence, rather than peace [84]. It is because of the combination of how one wants a conflict to end, versus mental health symptom, is has been suggested that psychotherapy should also concentrate on creating a sense justice in psychotherapy, not per say for the mental health issues, but for the post-war integration [85].

These findings related to terrorism studies in several ways. First, the importance of having shelter, food, and basic needs after terrorism. This confirms the basis of psychosocial care that will be shown in Chap. 9, namely people who experience trauma want to know where their family is and simply need to have their basic needs and questions met.

Second, if terrorism is a societal attack, it must have wider repercussions than just the attack itself. Indeed, it can cause fear, but also can have severe economic repercussions, as shown in Chap. 4. These economic repercussions are often not taken into account for terrorism survivors, despite the no doubt many such problems arising after the attacks, when, for example, the place of the attack was their place of work, or if their work is affected in any way.

Third, as in the section on state terror, justice is important here as well, but is also showcases that this sense of justice is related to mental health issues, indicating that if a society wants to heal after a terrorist attack, and wants to create a sense of justice, it will need to take into account the mental health of terrorism's victims.

**Children and Adolescents**

One group that is, similarly to terrorism, especially at risk of mental health issues, are children and adolescents [86]. In Syria, almost all Syrian school children had some form of exposure to violent events, and more than half suffered from PTSD. Almost one in three of Syrian students had PTSD during the civil war, and almost half of those who experienced sexual assault had PTSD [79, 87, 88]. The depression symptoms of internally displaced girls and young women were correlated with the number of trauma events they were exposed to, with almost half of them having experienced direct combat violence, and one third wanted to harm themselves [89].

A study in a war zone in Thailand showcased the difference between direct and indirect exposure in children. Direct exposure was much more related to, aside from mental health issues, behavioural problems [90].

However, there is also evidence of strong resilience even among minors. While roughly half of Bedouin Palestinian children seemed to suffer from PTSD [91], authors have also noted the strong adaptation of children to traumatic circumstances when they are able to rely on personal, familial and communal supports [92, 93].

This fits the critique often given on studies on terrorism's impact on children's mental health, namely that their resilience is much higher than one would expect based on the library of studies [94]. Indeed, there needs to be attention for their mental health, but also with children there is mental health.

**Veterans and Social Inclusion**

One observation in veterans of war that is relevant for terrorism is the notion that veterans often felt happier in war zones than at home. Or at least that is the observation in Sebastian Junger's book "Tribe" [95]. While his argument goes too far—in that adversity leads to more social cohesion is a very Western argument—what is important to take away from it is that the community is important, and also understanding in that community. Studies on veterans

(continued)

(continued)

have had a more dynamic approach, where social support is not just social support—it is those who understand, who can actually help. In terrorism research (and disaster research in general), the assumption is that any form of social support will do, yet studies also show that most social support gets tired of trying to help, or does not provide any real support because they do not understand what the person has gone through. Indeed, a book like "Tribe" showcases the message of the importance of community in getting through mental health issues after severe trauma. This will be showcased in Chap. 7 as well, where survivors of terrorism tend to seek out other survivors of terrorism, yet there is surprisingly little insight into those dynamics in civilians, while among veterans it is clear—and in fact, part of popular culture in terms of movies and books.

## 6.7 Migration

When refugees end up in detentions centres, the stress of past experiences and the stress of being in the detention centre have been associated with high PTSD rates, especially among children [96]. Syrian refugees displaced to nearby countries, such as Jordan, often reside in poverty, have no access to proper healthcare, and live in conditions where they are open to further trauma exposure [97]. Girls are, for example, open to gender-based violence and gender barriers in their access to education in host countries [98]. Additionally, studies among Syrian refugees in Lebanon also showed that refugees without legal residency status fear taking up any form of healthcare, out of fear of being deported [99].

However, mental health issues are also on average high among Syrian refugees living in Nordic countries [100, 101], especially among women and older refugees. One study in Sweden showed that PTSD rates were around 30% for Syrian refugees, and that in addition to pre-migration trauma exposure, there was substantial post-migration stress, due to everything associated with the migration process, administration, and adapting to a new culture, language, and climate [102–104]. The barriers also limit their access to healthcare [103, 104].

Studies on Syrian refugees in Turkey also showed that post-migration stress can include the fear of losing their ethnic identity, as well as fear of having nothing to fall back on [105].

Problems among refugees can also stay for a long time. Cambodian refugees after the civil war and genocide in Cambodia, even after two decades after resettlement, still suffered from high levels of PTSD, which was associated with being older, poor English proficiency, unemployment, poverty, etc [106]. Similarly, among Guatemalan refugees in Mexico, 20 years after fleeing for civil conflict, still show high percentages of PTSD (roughly 11%), and half had anxiety disorder, which was linked to having a high amount of exposure to traumatic events [107]. Finally, a study in Colombia, showed that among children who are internally displaced there is double as much PTSD as those not internally displaced, despite exposure to violence [108].

Such findings indicate that there are several elements of importance. First, as mentioned before, basic needs must be met, and stability is important. Secondly, as in terrorism studies, migrants indeed have many more difficulties in terms of mental health issues and accessing mental health care systems. In fact, very few terrorism studies have made the link between these migration studies and their own findings that indeed, migrants often are the biggest victims of terrorism, and the ones most often unable to access mental health care (see Chap. 8).

## 6.8 Living in Countries Near a War Zone

Living near war zones can also be associated with more mental health issues. For example, the war in Gaza was associated with more stress in the population in Jordan and Egypt [109–111]. This stress seems to be associated with, aside from the proximity of the attacks, historical reasons (e.g. the past wars of Israel) [112]. This is reflected also in the anxiety and depression noted in Poland, that is correlated with the war in Ukraine, but also the political and economic instability in Eastern Europe and the fear of Russia again controlling Poland [113–118].

So, while proximity is important [119], it certainly is not the only reason [120]. One study compared people in Ukraine, Poland, and Taiwan, and, while Ukrainians are most distressed, Taiwan people also are distressed due to images [121, 122]. This might be due to the historical dependency on the United States as protector against China, in which Ukraine might prove evidence of changing priorities of the United States.

As such, a difficulty in studies showcased in Chap. 4, that reviews studies on the impact of terrorism on society, is that such contextual factors seldom play a role, as well as other aspects. Indeed, a country that is politically instable might suffer more from a terrorist attack (or vice versa, for that matter), but due to a tunnel vision in terrorism studies, this is often not noticed, nor taken into account.

## 6.9 Reflections on Terrorism and Mental Health

Despite the difference between the events (one cliché says "If you have seen one disaster, you have seen one disaster"—indicating how idiosyncratic disasters are), there are certain reactions to these events that are similar to terrorism. For example, PTSD and depression as the most common reactions to violence. Studies also focus on similar risk groups, such as children and adolescents, while also looking at the association between proximity and PTSD.

However, major lessons can be learned from social aspects. First, the importance of community and social relationships is much more obvious in these types of studies than in studies on terrorism. This might be partly due to the strong focus in Western countries, where the majority of terrorism studies have been conducted, on the psychiatric lens: things need to be expressed in mental health terms [123–125], yet as the later chapter on social relationships will show, the importance of studying the community interactions after terrorist attacks is of the upmost importance for understanding how the community can be helped to recover, and how the community can help each other recover [27].

Secondly, these studies also show other risk factors. For example, a risk factor not often taken into account in terrorism studies is the loss of your home. Most terrorist attacks indeed do not affect the home of anyone, but they do often affect the workplace. Chapter 2 showed the relation between the workplace being targeted and how employees deal with the aftermath, but these are mainly based on 9/11, the Norway and the Brussels attacks.

Third, qualitative studies (e.g. interviews with survivors) are rare in terrorism research. This has, arguably, led the field into repetition of results. Most studies focus on PTSD, without much attention for how the political impact of such disasters are. As the studies in Myanmar showed, the war was one thing, but there was also an economic crisis and other mass stressor events taking place. Trauma is a lived reality, not a single data point; terrorism studies often have as focus one event and try to explain everything through that exposure.

This is not to say that other disaster studies are as broad oriented as perhaps indicated here; however, they are often forced to take other aspects of their topics into account because they are difficult to explain without doing so.

Fourth, justice and revenge are aspects seldom studied among survivors of terrorism, despite that it is clear that this has an important social role, and a clear relation with mental health, yet the sense of justice and the need for revenge would seem to be important in the aftermath of an attack on one's country. In fact, 9/11 led to two wars in the Middle East, yet few studies looked at the survivors' perspective of how their sense of justice related to these wars.

In short, other fields of disaster studies have, on the one hand, a lot of overlap with terrorism studies and, on the other hand, they have a lot to teach on terrorism studies—and no doubt, vice versa, but that is not the focus of this chapter.

## References


1. Drury J, Williams R. Children and young people who are refugees, internally displaced persons or survivors or perpetrators of war, mass violence and terrorism. Curr Opin Psychiatry. 2012;25:277–84.
2. Weisleder P, Rublee C. The neuropsychological consequences of armed conflicts and torture. Curr Neurol Neurosci Rep. 2018;18:9.
3. Shelef L, Schiff M, Pat-Horenczyk R, et al. COVID-19 vs. terrorism: contribution of the COR theory to the process of coping with invisible threats. J Psychiatr Res. 2022;147:176–82.
4. Ishtiaq H, Batool TE, Mamoon B, et al. Mental health problems in Pakistani society as a consequence of violence and trauma: a case for better integration of care. Cureus. 2025;17:e83486.

5. van der Velden PG, Contino C, Das M, et al. To what extent do post-traumatic mental health and other problems reflect pre-existing problems? Findings from the prospective comparative population-based VICTIMS-study. Int J Soc Psychiatry. 2023;69:841–52.
6. Golitaleb M, Mazaheri E, Bonyadi M, et al. Prevalence of post-traumatic stress disorder after flood: a systematic review and meta-analysis Front Psychiatry; 13. Epub ahead of print 23 June 2022. https://doi.org/10.3389/fpsyt.2022.890671.
7. Tahernejad S, Ghaffari S, Ariza-Montes A, et al. Post-traumatic stress disorder in medical workers involved in earthquake response: a systematic review and meta-analysis. Heliyon. 2023;9:e12794.
8. Tuturea LE, Narita ZC, Shimomura K, et al. Long-term mental health trajectories after the Great East Japan Earthquake: a systematic review. Eur J Psychotraumatol; 16. Epub ahead of print 31 December 2025. https://doi.org/10.1080/20008066.2025.2592408.
9. Bernstein M, Pfefferbaum B. Posttraumatic growth as a response to natural disasters in children and adolescents. Curr Psychiatry Rep. 2018;20:37.
10. Toper F, Yanardağ R, Koca M, et al. Post-traumatic growth in university students after earthquakes: the effect of perceived social support and psychological resilience. Behav Sci. 2025;15:1178.
11. Woods CF, McIntosh VVW, Beaglehole B, et al. Mental health service utilization after natural disasters: a systematic review. Epub ahead of print 9 January 2026. https://doi.org/10.1176/appi.ps.20250063.
12. Bustnes KA, Schäfer S, Held L, et al. Risks to the unborn: an umbrella review on the effects of prenatal maternal stress caused by natural disasters. Stress Health; 41. Epub ahead of print 28 October 2025. https://doi.org/10.1002/smi.70108.
13. Lee S, First JM. Mental health impacts of tornadoes: a systematic review. Int J Environ Res Public Health. 2022;19:13747.
14. Zortea TC, Kõlves K, Russell K, et al. Natural disasters and suicidal behaviour: an updated systematic review. J Affect Disord. 2025;375:256–92.
15. Hossain M, Talukder TT. A comprehensive review on post-wildfire impacts in California: environmental exposure, health risks, and resilience strategies. J Environ Sci Health A. 2025;60:468–84.
16. Aguilera R, Corringham T, Gershunov A, et al. Wildfire smoke impacts respiratory health more than fine particles from other sources: observational evidence from Southern California. Nat Commun. 2021;12:1493.
17. Dickinson N, Spencer LH, Yang S, et al. Extreme weather events in the UK and resulting public health outcomes. Int J Public Health; 70. Epub ahead of print 29 May 2025. https://doi.org/10.3389/ijph.2025.1607904.
18. Hartman CW, Squires GD. There is no such thing as a natural disaster: race, class, and Hurricane Katrina. Routledge; 2006.
19. Palgi Y, Dicker-Oren SD, Greene T. Evaluating a community fire as human-made vs. natural disaster moderates the relationship between peritraumatic distress and both PTSD symptoms and posttraumatic growth. Anxiety Stress Coping. 2020;33:569–80.
20. Jessica S. The ultimate terrorists. Harvard University Press; 2001.
21. Janoff-Bulman R. The aftermath of victimization: rebuilding shattered assumptions. In: Figley C, editor. Trauma and its wake. London: Routledge; 1985.
22. Pynchon T. V. Vintage, 1963.
23. Erikson K. Everything in its path: destruction of community in the Buffalo Creek Flood. Simon & Schuster; 1976.
24. Erikson K. Notes on trauma and community. In: Caruth C, editor. Trauma: explorations in memory. Hopkins University Press; 1995.
25. Felman S. Education and crisis, or the vicissitudes of teaching. In: Caruth C, editor. Exploration in memory. John Hopkins University Press; 1995.

26. Stein JY, Levin Y, Bachem R, et al. Growing apart: a longitudinal assessment of the relation between post-traumatic growth and loneliness among combat veterans. Front Psychol; 9. Epub ahead of print 7 June 2018. https://doi.org/10.3389/fpsyg.2018.00893.
27. Possick C, Shamai M, Sadeh RA. Healing the social self: how parents whose children were killed in terror attacks construct the experience of help. Community Ment Health J. 2014;50:487–96.
28. Muysewinkel E, Stene LE, Van Deynse H, et al. Post-what stress? A review of methods of research on posttraumatic stress during COVID-19. J Anxiety Disord. 2024;102:102829.
29. FORSTER JOHN. LIFE OF CHARLES DICKENS, VOLUME II: 1847-1870. COSIMO CLASSICS, 1874.
30. Harrington R. The railway accident: trains, trauma, and technoloigcal crises in nineteenth-century Britain. In: Traumatic pasts. Cambridge: Cambridge University Press; 2001.
31. Robert F. The whiplash encyclopedia : the facts and myths of whiplash. Aspen Publishers; 1999.
32. Harrington R. On the tracks of trauma: railway spine reconsidered. Social Hist Med. 2003;16:209–23.
33. Van Overmeire R, Muysewinkel E, Van Keer R-L, et al. Victims of the terrorist attacks in Belgium and professional mental health aid barriers: a qualitative study Front Psychiatry; 12. Epub ahead of print 2 July 2021. https://doi.org/10.3389/fpsyt.2021.638272.
34. Hazarika S. INDIAN JOURNALIST OFFERED WARNING. New York Times.
35. Tachakra S. The Bhopal disaster. J R Soc Health. 1987;107:1–2.
36. Rs M. Mental health of survivors of 1984 Bhopal disaster: a continuing challenge. Ind Psychiatry J. 2014;23:86.
37. Moussa S, El KM, Enaba D, et al. Impact of political violence on the mental health of school children in Egypt. J Ment Health. 2015;24:289–93.
38. Ni MY, Li TK, Pang H, et al. Longitudinal patterns and predictors of depression trajectories related to the 2014 occupy central/umbrella movement in Hong Kong. Am J Public Health. 2017;107:593–600.
39. Bi K, Chan CS, Xiao Y, et al. The indirect effect of sleep on the association between protracted social stressors and psychological distress among Hong Kong young people. J Adolesc Health. 2023;72:788–95.
40. Lai DWL, Ou X, Lee VWP, et al. Exposure to violence in social unrest, resilience, and mental health of older people in Hong Kong. Am J Geriatr Psychiatry. 2023;31:1091–9.
41. Glushkova N, Ivankov A, Trenina V, et al. Post-conflict acute stress reactions in Kazakhstan in the aftermath of January 2022 unrests: a national survey. Heliyon. 2023;9:e21065.
42. Ni MY, Kim Y, McDowell I, et al. Mental health during and after protests, riots and revolutions: a systematic review. Aust N Z J Psychiatry. 2020;54:232–43.
43. Levi-Belz Y, Groweiss Y, Blank C. Moral injury and its mental health consequences among protesters: findings from Israel's civil protest against the government's judicial reform. Eur J Psychotraumatol. 2023;14:2283306.
44. Griffin BJ, Purcell N, Burkman K, et al. Moral injury: an integrative review. J Trauma Stress. 2019;32:350–62.
45. Muysewinkel E, Vesentini L, Van Deynse H, et al. A day in the life: psychological impact on emergency responders during the 22 March 2016 terrorist attacks. Front Psychiatry; 15. Epub ahead of print 12 February 2024. https://doi.org/10.3389/fpsyt.2024.1353130.
46. Van Overmeire R, Van Keer R, Bilsen J. Impact of terrorist attacks on social relationships. Clin Psychol Psychother. 2021;28:1472–81.
47. Levi-Belz Y, Blank C, Groweiss Y, et al. The impact of potentially morally injurious experience of betrayal on PTSD and depression following the October 7th terror attack. Sci Rep. 2024;14:18021.
48. Diamond J. Upheaval: how nations cope with crisis and change. Penguin Books; 2019.
49. Beckert S. Capitalism: a global history. New York: Penguin Press; 2025.

50. Cárdenas Castro M, Arnoso Martínez M, Faúndez AX. Deliberate rumination and positive reappraisal as serial mediators between life impact and posttraumatic growth in victims of state terrorism in Chile (1973-1990). J Interpers Violence. 2019;34:545–61.
51. Steel Z, Chey T, Silove D, et al. Association of torture and other potentially traumatic events with mental health outcomes among populations exposed to mass conflict and displacement. JAMA. 2009;302:537.
52. Bendfeldt-Zachrisson F. Torture as intensive repression in Latin America: the psychology of its methods and practice. Int J Health Serv. 1988;18:301–10.
53. Cárdenas-Castro M, Faúndez-Abarca X, Arancibia-Martini H, et al. The relationship between posttraumatic growth and psychosocial variables in survivors of state terrorism and their relatives. J Interpers Violence. 2021;36:428–47.
54. Cárdenas M, Páez D, Rimé B, et al. Personal emotions, emotional climate, social sharing, beliefs, and values among people affected and unaffected by past political violence. Peace Conflict J Peace Psychol. 2014;20:452–64.
55. Cárdenas M, Páez D, Rimé B, et al. How transitional justice processes and official apologies influence reconciliation: the case of the Chilean 'Truth and Reconciliation' and 'Political Imprisonment and Torture' commissions. J Community Appl Soc Psychol. 2015;25:515–30.
56. Konvisser ZD. Themes of resilience and growth in survivors of politically motivated violence. Traumatology (Tallahass Fla). 2013;19:292–302.
57. Nilsen LG, Thoresen S, Wentzel-Larsen T, et al. Trust after terror: institutional trust among young terror survivors and their parents after the 22nd of July terrorist attack on Utøya Island, Norway. Front Psychol; 10. Epub ahead of print 13 December 2019. https://doi.org/10.3389/fpsyg.2019.02819.
58. Morina N, Stam K, Pollet TV, et al. Prevalence of depression and posttraumatic stress disorder in adult civilian survivors of war who stay in war-afflicted regions. A systematic review and meta-analysis of epidemiological studies. J Affect Disord. 2018;239:328–38.
59. Ghazy RM, Mohammed YY, Tolba B, et al. Prevalence and determinants of depression and anxiety among Sudanese during the ongoing civil conflicts: a cross-sectional study. Medicine. 2025;104:e41553.
60. Peconga EK, Høgh TM. Post-traumatic stress disorder, depression, and anxiety in adult Syrian refugees: what do we know? Scand J Public Health. 2020;48:677–87.
61. Tay AK. The mental health needs of displaced people exposed to armed conflict. Lancet Public Health. 2022;7:e398–9.
62. Seino K, Takano T, Mashal T, et al. Prevalence of and factors influencing posttraumatic stress disorder among mothers of children under five in Kabul, Afghanistan, after decades of armed conflicts. Health Qual Life Outcomes. 2008;6:29.
63. Ayazi T, Lien L, Eide A, et al. Association between exposure to traumatic events and anxiety disorders in a post-conflict setting: a cross-sectional community study in South Sudan. BMC Psychiatry. 2014;14:6.
64. Ayazi T, Lien L, Eide AH, et al. What are the risk factors for the comorbidity of posttraumatic stress disorder and depression in a war-affected population? A cross-sectional community study in South Sudan. BMC Psychiatry. 2012;12:175.
65. Xu W, Pavlova I, Chen X, et al. Mental health symptoms and coping strategies among Ukrainians during the Russia-Ukraine war in March 2022. Int J Soc Psychiatry. 2023;69:957–66.
66. Khan AR, Altalbe A. Potential impacts of Russo-Ukraine conflict and its psychological consequences among Ukrainian adults: the post-COVID-19 era. Front Public Health. 2023;11:1280423.
67. Birhan Z, Shegaw M, Kunno K, et al. Prevalence of suicidal behavior and its associated factors among individuals living in war-affected areas of Dessie Town, northeast Ethiopia, in 2022: a cross-sectional study. Front Psychiatry. 2025;16:1453526.

68. Tinsae T, Shumet S, Tadesse G, et al. Post-traumatic stress disorder in the Ethiopian population dwelling in war-affected communities: a systematic review and meta-analysis. Front Psychiatry. 2024;15:1399013.
69. Klarić M, Francisković T, Klarić B, et al. Social support and PTSD symptoms in war-traumatized women in Bosnia and Herzegovina. Psychiatr Danub. 2008;20:466–73.
70. Kliewer W, Fearnow MD, Miller PA. Coping socialization in middle childhood: tests of maternal and paternal influences. Child Dev. 1996;67:2339–57.
71. Griffith JL, Agani F, Weine S, et al. A family-based mental health program of recovery from state terror in Kosova. Behav Sci Law. 2005;23:547–58.
72. Hall BJ, Murray SM, Galea S, et al. Loss of social resources predicts incident posttraumatic stress disorder during ongoing political violence within the Palestinian Authority. Soc Psychiatry Psychiatr Epidemiol. 2015;50:561–8.
73. Kohrt BA, Hruschka DJ, Worthman CM, et al. Political violence and mental health in Nepal: prospective study. Br J Psychiatry. 2012;201:268–75.
74. Thapa SB, Hauff E. Psychological distress among displaced persons during an armed conflict in Nepal. Soc Psychiatry Psychiatr Epidemiol. 2005;40:672–9.
75. Luitel NP, Jordans MJD, Sapkota RP, et al. Conflict and mental health: a cross-sectional epidemiological study in Nepal. Soc Psychiatry Psychiatr Epidemiol. 2013;48:183–93.
76. Mesa-Vieira C, Haas AD, Buitrago-Garcia D, et al. Mental health of migrants with pre-migration exposure to armed conflict: a systematic review and meta-analysis. Lancet Public Health. 2022;7:e469–81.
77. Thapa SB, Hauff E. Perceived needs, self-reported health and disability among displaced persons during an armed conflict in Nepal. Soc Psychiatry Psychiatr Epidemiol. 2012;47:589–95.
78. Bendavid E, Boerma T, Akseer N, et al. The effects of armed conflict on the health of women and children. Lancet. 2021;397:522–32.
79. Yousef L, Ebrahim O, AlNahr MH, et al. War-related trauma and post-traumatic stress disorder prevalence among Syrian university students. Eur J Psychotraumatol. 2021;12:1954774.
80. Ahmed M, Yeddi AA, Alrawa SS, et al. Anxiety and depression symptoms among a sample of Khartoum civilians during the 2023 Sudan armed conflict: a cross-sectional study. PLoS One. 2023;19:e0307648.
81. Fan X, Ning K, Ma TSW, et al. Post-traumatic stress, depression, and anxiety during the 2021 Myanmar conflict: a nationwide population-based survey. Lancet Reg Health Southeast Asia. 2024;26:100396.
82. Avdibegović E, Hasanović M, Selimbasić Z, et al. Mental health care of psychotraumatized persons in post-war Bosnia and Herzegovina--experiences from Tuzla Canton. Psychiatr Danub. 2008;20:474–84.
83. Başoğlu M, Livanou M, Crnobarić C, et al. Psychiatric and cognitive effects of war in former Yugoslavia. JAMA. 2005;294:580.
84. Vinck P, Pham PN, Stover E, et al. Exposure to war crimes and implications for peace building in Northern Uganda. JAMA. 2007;298:543.
85. Kizilhan JI, Neumann J. The significance of justice in the psychotherapeutic treatment of traumatized people after war and crises Front Psychiatry; 11. Epub ahead of print 19 June 2020. https://doi.org/10.3389/fpsyt.2020.00540.
86. Uphoff E, Robertson L, Cabieses B, et al. An overview of systematic reviews on mental health promotion, prevention, and treatment of common mental disorders for refugees, asylum seekers, and internally displaced persons. Cochrane Database Syst Rev. 2020;9:CD013458.
87. Kakaje A, Al Zohbi R, Alyousbashi A, et al. Post-traumatic stress disorder (PTSD), anger and mental health of school students in Syria after nine years of conflict: a large-scale school-based study. Psychol Med. 2022;52:1923–33.
88. Perkins JD, Ajeeb M, Fadel L, et al. Mental health in Syrian children with a focus on post-traumatic stress: a cross-sectional study from Syrian schools. Soc Psychiatry Psychiatr Epidemiol. 2018;53:1231–9.

89. Pearson I, Chase E, Van Kim C, et al. Conflict exposure and mental health: a survey of adolescent girls and young women in Myanmar post the 2021 coup d'état. Confl Heal. 2025;19:29.
90. Jayuphan J, Sangthong R, Hayeevani N, et al. Mental health problems from direct vs indirect exposure to violent events among children born and growing up in a conflict zone of southern Thailand. Soc Psychiatry Psychiatr Epidemiol. 2020;55:57–62.
91. Massad S, Khammash U, Shute R. Political violence and mental health of Bedouin children in the West Bank, Palestine: a cross-sectional study. Med Confl Surviv. 2017;33:188–206.
92. Slone M, Peer A. Children's reactions to war, armed conflict and displacement: resilience in a social climate of support. Curr Psychiatry Rep. 2021;23:76.
93. Veronese G, Pepe A, Obaid H, et al. Agency and life satisfaction in Bedouin children exposed to conditions of chronic stress and military violence: a two-wave longitudinal study in Palestine. Clin Child Psychol Psychiatry. 2020;25:242–59.
94. Durodié B, Wainwright D. Terrorism and post-traumatic stress disorder: a historical review. Lancet Psychiatry. 2019;6:61–71.
95. Junger Sebastian. Tribe: on homecoming and belonging. 4th Estate, 2017.
96. Priestley I, Cherian S, Paxton G, et al. The impact of immigration detention on children's mental health: systematic review. Br J Psychiatry. 2025;227:870–9.
97. Al-Hourani D, Al-Wriekat M, Llamas-Ramos R, et al. The psychological impact among Syrian refugees in host countries. Healthcare (Basel); 13. Epub ahead of print 24 February 2025. https://doi.org/10.3390/healthcare13050488.
98. Hattar-Pollara M. Barriers to education of Syrian refugee girls in Jordan: gender-based threats and challenges. J Nurs Scholarsh. 2019;51:241–51.
99. Ragi M-E, Ghattas H, Abi Zeid B, et al. Legal residency status and its relationship with health indicators among Syrian refugees in Lebanon: a nested cross-sectional study. BMJ Glob Health; 10. Epub ahead of print 20 February 2025. DOI: 10.1136/bmjgh-2024-017767.
100. Ojha S, Thapa S, Thapa SB. Mental health problems among Syrian refugees in Nordic countries: a systematic review. Nord J Psychiatry. 2024;78:561–9.
101. Nissen A, Cauley P, Saboonchi F, et al. Mental health in adult refugees from Syria resettled in Norway between 2015 and 2017: a nationwide, questionnaire-based, cross-sectional prevalence study. Eur J Psychotraumatol. 2021;12:1994218.
102. Tinghög P, Malm A, Arwidson C, et al. Prevalence of mental ill health, traumas and postmigration stress among refugees from Syria resettled in Sweden after 2011: a population-based survey. BMJ Open. 2017;7:e018899.
103. Kiselev N, Pfaltz M, Schick M, et al. Problems faced by Syrian refugees and asylum seekers in Switzerland. Swiss Med Wkly. 2020;150:w20381.
104. Kiselev N, Pfaltz M, Haas F, et al. Structural and socio-cultural barriers to accessing mental healthcare among Syrian refugees and asylum seekers in Switzerland. Eur J Psychotraumatol. 2020;11:1717825.
105. Yilmaz E, Tamam L, Cengisiz C. Post-traumatic stress disorder among long-term resettled Syrian refugees in Turkey: a comprehensive analysis of pre- and post-migratory factors. Front Psychiatry. 2024;15:1352288.
106. Marshall GN, Schell TL, Elliott MN, et al. Mental health of Cambodian refugees 2 decades after resettlement in the United States. JAMA. 2005;294:571–9.
107. Sabin M, Lopes Cardozo B, Nackerud L, et al. Factors associated with poor mental health among Guatemalan refugees living in Mexico 20 years after civil conflict. JAMA. 2003;290:635–42.
108. Gómez-Restrepo C, Cruz-Ramírez V, Medina-Rico M, et al. Mental health in displaced children by armed conflict – National Mental Health Survey Colombia 2015. Actas Esp Psiquiatr. 2018;46:51–7.
109. Al-Ajlouny S, Al-Maqableh HO, Al-Shaikh AF, et al. Exploring the psychological effects of war on indirectly affected groups: a cross-sectional study on residents of Jordan. BMC Psychiatry. 2025;25:130.
110. Alhalaseh L, Alghzawi A, Khalifa S, et al. Unseen repercussions of war: psychological effects on Jordanians during the Israeli Palestinian war. Eur J Psychotraumatol. 2025;16:2506961.

111. Hendawy M, Abouzid M, Gamal A, et al. Psychological distress among students in Egypt and Jordan during the initial months of the Gaza war. BMC Psychol. 2024;12:678.
112. Shlaim A. The Iron Wall: Israel and the Arab world. Penguin; 2014.
113. Hisato T, Nandy S, Monga EM, et al. Psychological distress among healthcare students in Poland from COVID-19 to war on Ukraine: a cross-sectional exploratory study. Front Public Health. 2023;11:1186442.
114. Grzankowska I, Wójtowicz-Szefler M, Deja M. Selected determinants of anxiety and depression symptoms in adolescents aged 11-15 in relation to the pandemic COVID-19 and the war in Ukraine. Front Public Health. 2024;12:1480416.
115. Wójtowicz-Szefler M, Grzankowska I, Deja M. The mental condition of Polish adolescents during the COVID-19 pandemic and war in Ukraine. Front Public Health. 2023;11:1257384.
116. Błaszczyk Z, Wyrzychowski A, Plewka M, et al. Resilience of pregnant Polish women during the war between Ukraine and Russia. Sci Rep. 2025;15:16228.
117. Gambin M, Wnuk A, Oleksy T, et al. Depressive and anxiety symptom trajectories in Polish adolescents during the COVID-19 pandemic and the outbreak of war in Ukraine: uncovering the role of family relations. Dev Psychopathol. 2024;36:1948–58.
118. Barszcz E, Plewka M, Gajewska A, et al. Perinatal depression, labor anxiety and mental well-being of Polish women during the perinatal period in a war and economic crisis. Psychiatry. 2025;88:126–41.
119. Kalaitzaki A, Goodwin R, Kurapov A, et al. The mental health toll of the Russian-Ukraine war across 11 countries: cross-sectional data on war-related stressors, PTSD and CPTSD symptoms. Psychiatry Res. 2024;342:116248.
120. Greenglass ER, Begic P, Buchwald P, et al. Watching the Russian–Ukrainian war: comparison between Europe and North America. Behav Sci. 2025;15:1319.
121. Chudzicka-Czupała A, Hapon N, Chiang S-K, et al. Depression, anxiety and post-traumatic stress during the 2022 Russo-Ukrainian war, a comparison between populations in Poland, Ukraine, and Taiwan. Sci Rep. 2023;13:3602.
122. Chudzicka-Czupała A, Hapon N, Man RHC, et al. Associations between coping strategies and psychological distress among people living in Ukraine, Poland, and Taiwan during the initial stage of the 2022 War in Ukraine. Eur J Psychotraumatol. 2023;14:2163129.
123. Peter C. The medicalization of society: on the transformation of human conditions into treatable disorders. Johns Hopkins University Press; 2007.
124. Horwitz AVV. PTSD: a short history. Johns Hopkins University Press; 2018.
125. Horwitz AV, Wakefield JC. The loss of sadness: how psychiatry transformed normal sorrow into depressive disorder. Oxford University Press; 2007.

# Chapter 7
# Stand by Me: Social Relationships After Terrorist Attacks

## 7.1 Introduction

Experiencing terrorism is deeply linked with social aspects. As Herman writes in her landmark work Trauma and Recovery, "*Recovery can take place only within the context of relationships; it cannot occur in isolation*" [1]. Indeed, mental health issues can be limited through the support one gets from their friends and family, or the risk can be higher when there is no support; the issues can be limited through the acknowledgement of what one is going through, or can be worsened because the experience is denied, and for the mental health aid that can be provided, the community is important.

In fact, the importance of social aspects is what has been called the paradox in post-traumatic stress disorder (PTSD): despite the many biological and psychological aspects to it, it is social support that is the best aid for those who develop PTSD [2]. Indeed, social relationships are found to be more important than any psychological intervention in helping survivors after trauma [3], while the quality of social relationships is a better predictor for mental health than biological or economic factors [4]. Social relationships themselves are generally divided into three categories [4]:

1. Social network
2. Social connectedness
3. Social support

Social network is the most straightforward: this is the view on the social ties one has, the number of people one knows, etc. It is the network around an individual that is being studied in relation to that individual [4, 5]. Social connectedness is the way a person experiences a sense of belonging inside a social relationship [6]. Both social networks and social relationships are both connected with improved outcomes for mental health [5–9].


R. Van Overmeire, *Terrorism, Mental Health and Aftercare*,
https://doi.org/10.1007/978-3-032-31560-1_7

However, the overwhelming number of studies have been on the last concept: social support. This will be discussed in the following section.

## 7.2 Social Support as a Concept

Social support as a concept has several approaches to understanding it. There are, roughly, three major dimensions [10]:

1. Enacted social support
2. Structural support
3. Perceived social support

Enacted (or received) social support is the actual action the support takes to aid another person, while structural social support is the size of the support network [10]. Perceived social support is the perception of someone of how much support is available, and how useful that support is to them [10].

This perceived social support is the most common studied form of social support [11]. The reason being, among other reasons, it can be easily studied through self-report questionnaires. For example, while social network studies would need more than one respondent, and social connectedness perhaps a qualitative approach (e.g. interview), perceived social support can be measured through a few questions. For example, a popular measuring scale of perceived social support is the Oslo Social Support scale, which has only three questions: one on how many people they can count on if they would have personal problems; another on how much interest people show in what the respondent does; and how easy they would get help from neighbors if they needed it [12]. As self-report questionnaires are cheaper than large studies on social ties, and the questionnaires for respondents are generally meant to be short, self-perceived social support is a popular concept in terrorism studies, where speed and costs are of the essence—especially shortly after an attack.

Perceived social support scales have become an almost equally common measurement as PTSD in trauma studies. In fact, it is almost idiosyncratic to not measure perceived social support in a self-report study, as if the researcher has not taken into account the social aspect of trauma. An important reason for this is that social support has consistently been associated with PTSD: the more perceived social support, the lower the PTSD (and vice versa). Multiple large-scale reviews have shown that perceiving more social support is associated with lower PTSD and vice versa: having no social support is associated with an increased PTSD risk [13, 14]. This is also the case for terrorism studies, that whether after 9/11 [15], Paris-attacks [16] or Norway [11], have found a positive association between social support and PTSD. Such results have made it into an almost mandatory indicator to take into account when measuring PTSD.

As perceived social support is the most studied indicator, in the following sections the findings will be explored more. First, it is important to differentiate between pre-terrorism perceived social support and post-terrorism perceived social support.

### 7.2.1 Pre-terrorism Perceived Social Support

The social support that people perceive *before* they are exposed to trauma [17] is one of the most important buffers against mental health issues after the trauma, while feeling no support means a much higher risk for the development of PTSD [18–20]. This is also true for terrorism. Meaning: if survivors had the feeling of having a lot of social support before the terrorist attacks took place, this effected the risk of getting PTSD afterwards.

For example, several studies in Israel showed that the social support one perceived before terrorist attacks was a buffer against depression or PTSD [21–23].

### 7.2.2 Post-terrorism Perceived Social Support

Perceived social support is also important as buffer *after* a terrorist attack. This was for example found in studies in Norway [24], where it was protective against PTSD, or in a long-term follow-up after 9/11, which showed positive effects of such social support against the development of depression and anxiety [25]. Similarly, 14 to 15 years after 9/11, low perceived social support after 9/11 predicted more depression and PTSD [15, 26]. Interestingly, these 9/11 studies also show that the "effect" goes both ways. Having PTSD roughly five to six years after 9/11, predicted having lower social support ten years later, and PTSD ten year after 9/11 predicted lower social support fourteen to fifteen years later [15].

Yet, a cohort study a few years after 9/11 showed that social support might lose its importance over time in community disasters [27]; indeed, other studies after more than a decade after 9/11 showed that social support indeed predicted lower depression, but not lower PTSD [28]. Then again, social support is related to self-efficacy, which in turn protects against PTSD. It might therefore be that the role of social support as buffer against PTSD is indirect [28]. Meaning: social support might not directly help with PTSD in the long run, but it might actually help the survivor get control over their life again, and in that way protect against PTSD.

## 7.3 Barriers in Social Support

That being said, another reason why social support might lose its protective effect over time might have to do with the actual help survivors receive. It is possible that they feel that support is there for them, while as the years go by, their perception of the support changes because the survivors see that the people they thought they could count on, let them down [10, 29, 30].

This would explain the stark difference in the result between studied on perceived social support, that see clear results, showcasing that perceived social support protects against PTSD and other mental health issues, while the results for enacted (or received) social support are mixed at best [11]. Meaning that while people might perceive that they have a lot of social support available, in practice, the provided support might not be that helpful; in fact, it might be even damaging [10].

One important aspect of this is the honeymoon period [31]. When an attack, or trauma, occurs, the survivors receive a lot of social support. There is a lot of empathy, understanding, and aid from their family, friends, and community. This is the so-called honeymoon period.

However, as time goes on, the support expects the survivor to move on, or has difficulty accepting the new situation, or other reasons. As one person who lost someone in a non-terrorist incident stated:

> *"…but as far as support goes; everyone says 'if I can do anything for you', but they don't offer again. This is what they say in that first couple of weeks, but once the funeral has been no-one comes and knocks on the door 'what do you want me to do?'"* [32]

As one survivor of the Brussels attacks stated:

> *"The (participant's name) who went away on 22 March 2016, he never came back home. That's someone else. And I do my best. But I will never be who I was before. My wife thinks that's annoying—when we fight, I say 'You'll have to accept it'."* [33]

Social support has to, by definition, occur in transaction with people [11]. As such, there are two, *not* mutually exclusive, reasons why social support might fail in having a buffering effect in the long-term: the survivor does not want the social support, or the family and friends do not want to provide social support anymore.

### *7.3.1 The Survivor Turns Social Support Away*

First, the survivor turns the social support away, because they feel the social support is unable to understand what the survivor has gone through [11]. A common issue among survivors of trauma is that "the others" are unable to understand what the experience was to the survivor. As one survivor of terrorism stated:

> *"I was completely locked in, because I was afraid, totally afraid. And (my husband) was afraid of losing his family. So, the attacks hit us in another way. Because we were divided. That was the most difficult part. Because my husband did not experience the explosion. He had no idea what we had been through and had seen. […] No one can imagine. No one can understand. Not even my husband. He was hurt in a way. And that wasn't very helpful. […] I expected too much of him. He felt alone. And I had expected too much of him, pushed him too much. I wanted to force him, but he could not. […] He often said 'I wish I was there with you, so we could have been together'"* [33].

Similarly, after the Manchester Arena bombing, family and friends were perceived to be unable to understand the experiences [34]. In fact, studies show that the feeling that others cannot understand what the survivor has gone through is not uncommon. After the Utoya attacks, around 20% of female survivors, and roughly

17% of male survivors agreed with the statement "Those who weren't at Utøya Island, wouldn't understand me" [11].

Related to this, it might also be that the survivor perceives that the support is tired of hearing it. For example, in one study on the Utoya attacks, 14% of the female survivors did not want to overburden their friends [11]. As such, the survivor might stay quiet and stop sharing their experience with the social support [11, 33]. This is also why someone can perceive high social support, but not use it because of the social support barriers they experience. As such: high *perceived* social support can occur with no *enacted* social support [11].

Secondly, stigma plays a big role in pushing social support away. For example, a mother who survived an attack was afraid of losing her social role as mother to her child due to the attack [33], or, for example, survivors of the Mumbai attacks had to take up new social roles, due to the loss of family members who were providing the income for the family, but after taking up these social roles, they often started isolating themselves from their community, out of shame, lack of time, or other reasons [35].

As such, survivors who do develop mental health issues, at times try to ignore their symptoms or deal with them on their own—with varying degrees of success [36–38]. Silence is therefore often the strategy of survivors who feel this barrier [33]. In fact, as one study found, what helps for such survivors who would have difficulties talking about their experiences is alcohol (which in turn increases their perceived social support) [39].

Third, a common reaction is also that the survivor pushes the social support away not due to a feeling of not being understood, or the fear of losing their normal life, but because of mental health reactions [40]. People with PTSD or depression sometimes push people away due to their mental health issues, or due to their changed behaviour, or affected social skills [11, 41]. As one study before and after 9/11 showed, anxiety predicated the loss of support *after* the attacks [42].

In general, the perception of those with a mental disorder is affected, and in addition, they can experience bouts of anger, aggressive behavior, chronic depression, etc. As one survivor stated:

> *"I trust people less. I do not have a lot of friends anymore. And I do not come outside. I mostly see my family. My sister, now and again. My brother. My son. My mother. That's about it ...".* [33]

Indeed, studies after the Bali attacks also showed that having mental health issues decreases the belief in social support [40], or as a survivor of the Manchester Arena bombing stated

> *"... That made it [distress] worse ... she wasn't a mum to me at that point, it was a good 6 months where she was my mum, but she wasn't being a mother ... but at the time, she didn't see what was happening, like I did blame her a lot for a lot of it ..."* [36]

### 7.3.2 Social Support Turns Away from the Survivor

However, the social support might also turn away from the survivors. There are many possible causes. The support might have their own problems to deal with (for example, they might have to deal with the loss of someone in the attacks on their own) [32], or they might feel overburdened by the issues of the survivor, or they have no understanding for the problems the survivor goes through [33]. As one survivor of the Brussels attacks stated:

> *"One of my friends said, 'Come on, it's been two years, do victims still need support?' And I think, you'd have to experience it yourself. How would you react? But I'm not going to fight over it. I just do not talk with that person about it anymore—if that's his opinion ... Maybe that's an ostrich tactic, but we have known each other so long, and we support each other—but not in this ... Fine."* [33]

A parent who lost their child in terrorism experienced the following:

> *"They don't like to hear how bad we have it. They want to hear how well we are doing and I think you do have to voice how bad we have it...One used to call a lot and ask me 'what's up?' And every time it [the answer] was 'O.K.'. Then one day simply she asked 'what's up?' and I told her truly what was up. Since then she doesn't call anymore..."* [43]

An important part of mental health issues is the invisibility of them: it is for many people difficult to understand that despite being uninjured physically, they would experience such consequences on a mental level from an attack [36]. In fact, survivors can feel neglected precisely because they do not have a physical injury of the attack, yet still suffer from its consequences [36].

People might blame the survivor for having been at the scene of the trauma, or for not recovering fast enough, or for being different due to traumatic experience [10]. One survivor stated:

> *"I do not see anyone anymore ... A colleague-friend of mine that I had known my whole career, she just stopped keeping in touch. Because they feel that's it's been long enough, people judge themselves when it has to stop. They see it more as an act than 'This is the time I need because of all those problems'. I could not understand that. Because she was a colleague-friend I had known my whole ... Well, sixteen years. And then she suddenly turned on me."* [33]

Such social reactions might explain the findings after 9/11: depression among survivors was not linked directly with the exposure, but with events following the attacks [28]. Indeed, in other fields the idea of secondary traumatization, due to, for example, reactions of others, has been noted. In fact, such negative social support might explain mental health issues better than positive social support [44].

### 7.3.3 Social Acknowledgement

However, the problem can be also viewed with a wider lens: the community and society at large. For example, as one survivor from the Manchester Arena bombing stated:

> *"Facebook was very brutal and very nasty. Just people making comments that were not very understanding and putting really horrible stuff that kinda worsened me"* [36].

This relates to something called "social acknowledgement," namely, how the community and society react to the trauma also matters. That is important, as social support refers to the people one knows, but it might be that society also has reactions to the trauma [29, 30].

This societal reaction might explain partly why sometimes trauma itself, even when there are no symptoms, is not disclosed or mentioned to others. For example, a nationally representative study in Belgium showed that 17.1% who experienced sexual assault never mentioned it to anyone—not even friends [14]. In fact, such overarching cultural factors could also explain why perhaps women are less able to address social support after trauma and suffer more consequences from trauma than men—though results remain conflicting on this [11].

Naturally, terrorism is a public trauma, in the sense that everyone knows it happened; the lack of disclosure can therefore be perhaps due to the stigma on mental health in society, which would also explain the silence about the trauma among some survivors of terrorism [33]. In fact, it has been noted that survivors of terrorism sometimes are shamed for suffering mental health issues, and are ostracized for it [33, 45]:

> *"It had become such a taboo topic. Which I found terrible, because I wanted to know what my colleagues had done that day. I knew they were there, and I wanted to talk about it with those that wanted to talk. But the only way you could do it anymore, was to somehow make sure you were alone with them, because if there were others, they were like 'Are you still nagging about that?' Even the head-officer, the head of the airport, said 'The act can stop now'. [...] And the head of human resources, he apparently said stuff like 'Those profiteers, that stay home!'"* [33]

## 7.4 New Social Support

By now, it is clear that social support is not as straightforward as it is being measured in so many studies. Indeed, social support cannot be caught in one single measure or concept, and overall, the mechanism behind social support remains poorly understood [11]. In fact, what complicates research even further is the creation of new social support in the aftermath of terrorism, or in the aftermath of the experience of the barriers mentioned before.

Survivors who, for whatever reason, cannot rely on their old social support tend to seek out those with similar experiences as them. Parents who lost their child in terrorist attacks reported how they lost their friends, but also sought out other parents who had lost their child in terrorist attacks. As one survivor explained:

> "*I mostly talked with colleagues. People who went through it, whether or not from a different perspective. Because it's difficult to explain the nuances to people who did not experience it. Not because they do not understand, but because you do not know how to put it into words … If you explain that in the ceiling of the terminal, there were body parts hanging around … You cannot even begin to comprehend that.*" [33]

In fact, researchers who interview people who experience a severe trauma or tragedy note that the interviewees are often happy and eager to talk about what they have gone through, as they often feel they cannot talk about it anymore [32]. Not surprisingly therefore, survivors seek out other survivors for support, so that they can keep talking about it with people who understand their experience, and whom they will not overburden with repeating their experiences.

As noted in non-terrorism studies, those traumatized tend to in, a first phase, seek support from friends and family, and in a second phase, when they feel they need to keep talking about the events, they seek out more structured social support: support groups, for example, or buddy groups [32, 34, 46–48]. In addition to providing social support, this structured form also is related to seeking out professional mental health aid more regularly [49].

Such structured social support can however also have a downside when they are not tailored to specific needs [32, 46–48]. When they are not, they might lead to the earlier mentioned barriers. In fact, there is even an added danger here, namely the creation of a so-called trauma membrane [50]. Despite its somewhat off-putting name, the concept refers to the danger that people are bonded by their trauma, and bonded by *reliving* their trauma over and over, in endless conversations that center on that trauma, while creating a wall (or "membrane") between those who experienced the trauma and those who did not [50].

This relates to the concept introduced in natural disaster studies (and discussed in Chap. 6), but is unfortunately missing in terrorism-studies: collective trauma [51, 52]. While people might lose their social connections they had before a disaster, they connect with those who also experienced the disaster. That sense of being understood is often what creates new social ties. These "co-experiencers" give the survivor a sense of belonging; or, to refer back to one of the concepts of the beginning of this chapter: social connectedness [33, 50, 53]. In fact, that is the major difference between survivors of disasters and from interpersonal violence: disaster survivors can have a collective trauma, and share the experiences, and avoid the stigma of talking about it to other survivors, while survivors of sexual assault or interpersonal violence often have to fear social exclusion or victim blaming [31].

## 7.5 Moving On

This chapter has shown that social relationships are not undamaged after terrorist attacks. There is, on the one hand, how one perceives their social support, and on the other hand the actual social support. This last form is where the issues can arise, where barriers come up, and where relationships can fall apart, yet at the same time, the chapter highlighted the transformative power of social relationships, finding new people, creating new bonds. Furthermore, the chapter showed that terrorism, while it might affect one person in a community, still affects a community as a whole—or at the very least, a family.

As such, it seems clear that public health interventions should not focus on trying to deliver so many psychological interventions to individuals. In fact, this chapter indicates that it would be better to use public health intervention to focus on creating social support in families and communities [33, 54–56]. Despite all nuances in this chapter, it remains clearly the best protection against mental health issues.

## 7.6 To End

Caruth [57] has described trauma as "*the confrontation with an event that, in its unexpectedness or horror, cannot be placed within the schemes of prior knowledge – that cannot, as George Bataille says, become a matter of 'intelligence' – and thus continually returns, in its exactness, at a later time.*" The DSM-IV had a similar description for trauma as "*an event outside the range of the usual human experience*" [58], while Herman [1] described trauma as an overwhelming force that leaves people helpless, as an event that "*overwhelms the ordinary systems of care that give people a sense of control, connection, and meaning.*"

It should not surprise that often the experience of someone who experiences trauma is difficult to understand for those who have not shared that experience. As such, terrorism exposure can never just be related to a mental health problem; it is a social problem.

## References

1. Herman J. Trauma and recovery. New York: Basic Books; 1992.
2. Maercker A. The paradox of the biopsychological and sociocultural levels in post-traumatic stress disorder. World Psychiatry. 2025;24:87–8.
3. Holt-Lunstad J, Smith TB, Layton JB. Social relationships and mortality risk: a meta-analytic review. PLoS Med. 2010;7:e1000316.
4. Santini ZI, Koyanagi A, Tyrovolas S, et al. The association between social relationships and depression: a systematic review. J Affect Disord. 2015;175:53–65.
5. Smith KP, Christakis NA. Social networks and health. Annu Rev Sociol. 2008;34:405–29.

6. Townsend KC, McWhirter BT. Connectedness: a review of the literature with implications for counseling, assessment, and research. J Couns Dev. 2005;83:191–201.
7. Wickramaratne PJ, Yangchen T, Lepow L, et al. Social connectedness as a determinant of mental health: a scoping review. PLoS One. 2022;17:e0275004.
8. Soares AKS, Goedert MCF, Vargas AF. Mental health and social connectedness during the COVID-19 pandemic: an analysis of sports and E-sports players. Front Psychol. 2022;13 https://doi.org/10.3389/fpsyg.2022.802653.
9. Oberle E, Ji XR, Alkawaja M, et al. Connections matter: adolescent social connectedness profiles and mental well-being over time. J Adolesc. 2024;96:31–48.
10. Zalta AK, Tirone V, Orlowska D, et al. Examining moderators of the relationship between social support and self-reported PTSD symptoms: a meta-analysis. Psychol Bull. 2021;147:33–54.
11. Thoresen S, Jensen TK, Wentzel-Larsen T, et al. Social support barriers and mental health in terrorist attack survivors. J Affect Disord. 2014;156:187–93.
12. Kocalevent R-D, Berg L, Beutel ME, et al. Social support in the general population: standardization of the Oslo social support scale (OSSS-3). BMC Psychol. 2018;6:31.
13. Wang Y, Chung MC, Wang N, et al. Social support and posttraumatic stress disorder: a meta-analysis of longitudinal studies. Clin Psychol Rev. 2021;85:101998.
14. Muysewinkel E, Vesentini L, Van Deynse H, et al. trauma exposure, social support and mental health in the general population in Belgium. Eur J Investig Health Psychol Educ. 2024;14:2047–56.
15. Liu SY, Li J, Leon LF, et al. The bidirectional relationship between posttraumatic stress symptoms and social support in a 9/11-Exposed Cohort: a longitudinal cross-lagged analysis. Int J Environ Res Public Health. 2022;19:2604.
16. Berthail B, Trousselard M, Lecouvey G, et al. Differences in predictive factors for post-traumatic stress disorder encompassing partial PTSD and full PTSD: a cross-sectional study among individuals exposed to the November 13, 2015 Paris attacks. Front Psychiatry. 2024;15 https://doi.org/10.3389/fpsyt.2024.1351695.
17. Butler LD, Morland LA, Leskin GA. Psychological Resilience in the Face of Terrorism. In: Psychology of terrorism. Oxford University Press; 2006. p. 400–17.
18. Drogendijk AN, van der Velden PG, Gersons BPR, et al. Lack of perceived social support among immigrants after a disaster: comparative study. Br J Psychiatry. 2011;198:317–22.
19. van der Velden PG, Contino C, Marchand M, et al. Does pre-event lack of emotional support increase the risk of post-event PTSD, anxiety, depression symptoms and lack of support? A comparative population-based study among victims of threat and violence. J Anxiety Disord. 2020;75:102269.
20. van der Velden PG, Komproe I, Contino C, et al. Which groups affected by Potentially Traumatic Events (PTEs) are most at risk for a lack of social support? A prospective population-based study on the 12-month prevalence of PTEs and risk factors for a lack of post-event social support. PLoS One. 2020;15:e0232477.
21. Shahar G, Henrich CC. Perceived family social support buffers against the effects of exposure to rocket attacks on adolescent depression, aggression, and severe violence. J Fam Psychol. 2016;30:163–8.
22. Henrich CC, Shahar G. Social support buffers the effects of terrorism on adolescent depression: findings from Sderot, Israel. J Am Acad Child Adolesc Psychiatry. 2008;47:1073–6.
23. Shahar G, Cohen G, Grogan KE, et al. Terrorism-related perceived stress, adolescent depression, and social support from friends. Pediatrics. 2009;124:e235–40.
24. Dyb G, Jensen TK, Nygaard E, et al. Post-traumatic stress reactions in survivors of the 2011 massacre on Utøya Island, Norway. British Journal of Psychiatry. 2014;204:361–7.
25. Pijnenburg LJ, Velikonja T, Pietrzak RH, et al. Perceived social support and longitudinal trajectories of depression and anxiety in World Trade Center responders. Soc Psychiatry Psychiatr Epidemiol. 2024;59:1413–24.

26. Jacobson MH, Norman C, Nguyen A, et al. Longitudinal determinants of depression among World Trade Center Health Registry enrollees, 14–15 years after the 9/11 attacks. J Affect Disord. 2018;229:483–90.
27. Adams RE, Boscarino JA. Predictors of PTSD and delayed PTSD after disaster. J Nerv Ment Dis. 2006;194:485–93.
28. Adams SW, Bowler RM, Russell K, et al. PTSD and comorbid depression: social support and self-efficacy in World Trade Center tower survivors 14–15 years after 9/11. Psychol Trauma. 2019;11:156–64.
29. Maercker A, Müller J. Social acknowledgment as a victim or survivor: a scale to measure a recovery factor of PTSD. J Trauma Stress. 2004;17:345–51.
30. Maercker A, Horn AB. A socio-interpersonal perspective on PTSD: the case for environments and interpersonal processes. Clin Psychol Psychother. 2013;20:465–81.
31. Maercker A, Hecker T. Broadening perspectives on trauma and recovery: a socio-interpersonal view of PTSD. Eur J Psychotraumatol. 2016;7 https://doi.org/10.3402/ejpt.v7.29303.
32. Aoun SM, Breen LJ, Rumbold B, et al. Matching response to need: what makes social networks fit for providing bereavement support? PLoS One. 2019;14:e0213367.
33. Van Overmeire R, Van Keer R, Bilsen J. Impact of terrorist attacks on social relationships. Clin Psychol Psychother. 2021;28:1472–81.
34. Drury J, Stancombe J, Williams R, et al. Survivors' experiences of informal social support in coping and recovering after the 2017 Manchester Arena bombing. BJPsych Open. 2022;8:e124.
35. Joseph J, Jaswal S. Psychosocial framework for understanding psychological distress among survivors of the November 26, 2008 Mumbai terror attack: beyond traumatic experiences and emergency medical care. Prehosp Disaster Med. 2014;29:330–8.
36. Stancombe J, Williams R, Drury J, et al. People's experiences of distress and psychosocial care following a terrorist attack: interviews with survivors of the Manchester Arena bombing in 2017. BJPsych Open. 2022;8:e41.
37. Lee S, First JM. Mental health impacts of tornadoes: a systematic review. Int J Environ Res Public Health. 2022;19:13747.
38. Van Overmeire R, Muysewinkel E, Van Keer R-L, et al. Victims of the terrorist attacks in belgium and professional mental health aid barriers: a qualitative study. Front Psychiatry. 2021;12 https://doi.org/10.3389/fpsyt.2021.638272.
39. Kane JC, Rapaport C, Zalta AK, et al. Regular drinking may strengthen the beneficial influence of social support on depression: findings from a representative Israeli sample during a period of war and terrorism. Drug Alcohol Depend. 2014;140:175–82.
40. Stevens GJ, Dunsmore JC, Agho KE, et al. Coping support factors among Australians affected by terrorism: 2002 Bali bombing survivors speak. Med J Aust. 2013;199:772–5.
41. Kaniasty K, Norris FH. Longitudinal linkages between perceived social support and posttraumatic stress symptoms: sequential roles of social causation and social selection. J Trauma Stress. 2008;21:274–81.
42. Farach FJ, Mennin DS, Smith RL, et al. The impact of pretrauma analogue GAD and posttraumatic emotional reactivity following exposure to the September 11 terrorist attacks: a longitudinal study. Behav Ther. 2008;39:262–76.
43. Possick C, Shamai M, Sadeh RA. Healing the social self: how parents whose children were killed in terror attacks construct the experience of help. Community Ment Health J. 2014;50:487–96.
44. Brewin CR, Holmes EA. Psychological theories of posttraumatic stress disorder. Clin Psychol Rev. 2003;23:339–76.
45. Van Overmeire R, Vesentini L, Van Keer R-L, et al. Working experiences of airport employees after a terrorist attack in Belgium: a qualitative study. Int J Dis Risk Reduct. 2021;64:102515.
46. Aoun SM, Breen LJ, White I, et al. What sources of bereavement support are perceived helpful by bereaved people and why? Empirical evidence for the compassionate communities approach. Palliat Med. 2018;32:1378–88.

47. Dyregrov K. Experiences of social networks supporting traumatically bereaved. OMEGA: J Death Dying. 2006;52:339–58.
48. Riley SG, Pettus KI, Abel J. The buddy group—peer support for the bereaved. London J Prim Care (Abingdon). 2018;10:68–70.
49. Pirard P, Motreff Y, Stene LE, et al. Initiation of multiple-session psychological care in civilians exposed to the November 2015 Paris terrorist attacks. Arch Public Health. 2023;81:207.
50. Austin LS, Godleski LS. Therapeutic approaches for survivors of disaster. Psychiatr Clin N Am. 1999;22:897–910.
51. Erikson K. Notes on trauma and community. In: Caruth C, editor. Trauma: explorations in memory. Hopkins University Press; 1995.
52. Erikson K. Everything in its path: destruction of community in the Buffalo Creek flood. Simon & Schuster; 1976.
53. Gagin R, Cohen M, Peled-Avram M, et al. An ongoing, multi-faceted program for victims of terror attacks and their families. Int J Emerg Ment Health. 2007;9:193–200.
54. Shalev AY. Further lessons from 9/11: does stress equal trauma? Psychiatry Interpersonal Biol Process. 2004;67:174–7.
55. Simon JB, Murphy JJ, Smith SM. Understanding and fostering family resilience. Fam J. 2005;13:427–36.
56. Walsh F. Family resilience: a framework for clinical practice. Fam Process. 2003;42:1–18.
57. Caruth C. Trauma and experience. In: Caruth C, editor. Trauma: explorations in memory. John Hopkins University; 1995.
58. American Psychiatric Association. Diagnostic and statistical manual of mental disorders. 4th ed; 1994.

# Chapter 8
# Trauma and Recovery: Barriers in Seeking Out Professional Mental Health Aid

## 8.1 Introduction

After the attack, the tending to wounds begins, which for some survivors is either partly or completely of a mental nature. As mentioned throughout, a minority of survivors of terrorism develop issues such as post-traumatic stress disorder (PTSD), depression, or anxiety [1–4]. However, the finding of professional aid for these mental health issues is often a struggle in itself, which is evident from the fact that the majority of people who would benefit from professional mental health aid do not actively reach out to it [5].

Indeed, across all disaster studies, an observation can be made that only a minority of disaster victims that need aid, receive it [6]. This is an observation that holds true across all types of healthcare system, whether the United States, Norway, or Paris: survivors of terrorism have unmet professional mental health care needs [7–9].

The question is then: why? Why do people who suffer from mental health issues do not seek professional mental health aid. The reason is not due to financial reasons—even in the United States, financial barriers are seldom the reason for not seeking out aid [10].

This chapter will provide an overview of the barriers that can be faced by survivors of terrorism when seeking professional mental health aid.


R. Van Overmeire, *Terrorism, Mental Health and Aftercare*,
https://doi.org/10.1007/978-3-032-31560-1_8

## 8.2 Factors Associated with Unmet Mental Health Aid

### *8.2.1 Background Factors Are an Important Indicator of Unmet Needs*

There are many different background factors that can be important, such as education level, gender and age. For example, after 9/11, background factors that even after 14 to 15 years later were important were race, age, and education level, wherein white and Hispanic people, higher educated people, and those who were younger sought aid soonest after 9/11 [11]. African Americans and Asian American were less likely to seek out mental health aid [10, 11].

Some studies also suggest that women tend to use mental health services more. For example, studies in Oslo showed that while female survivors only used 12% mental health services the year before the attacks, this became 73% the first year after the attacks. Among male survivors the pre-attack mental healthcare use was 7%, and went up to 61% a year later [12]. However, for both genders this decreased by the third year: 40% for females and 31% in males [12]. Similarly, in Norway, while primary healthcare usage increased in fathers and mothers after the attack, only mothers had a significant increase in use of specialized mental healthcare [13]. These differences between men and women are also evident in studies after the Bali attacks, where women were more pro-government outreach, while men were more inclined to help themselves [14], while 1 year after 9/11, medication use was higher among younger women than among men [15].

An additional factor is the survivor's prior experience with professional mental health aid. For example, 6 months after 9/11, there was a severe unmet need among survivors, who did not receive any aid, with one of the important indicators being that these survivors had no previous experience in getting to mental health [16, 17]. This was even still a predictor 14 to 15 years later [11].

The reverse is also true: the best predictor for seeking out mental health aid was previous experience [11, 16]. It might be that having a pre-established knowledge of the mental health care system is important [11, 18]. Studies from Belgium show that even in accessible mental health care systems, it is a search for mental health aid, as well as knowing the way to reimburse it [19]. Furthermore, a prior relationship with a healthcare provider allows the barrier to seek out help to be lower [11, 18].

### *8.2.2 Not Being Injured Physically*

Studies in Belgium show that those without physical injuries often had more difficulties getting reimbursements from the government for suffered injuries and also realizing that they had to seek out mental health aid for their injuries [19]. Compared to physically uninjured people, injured people often have the possibility to talk to hospital staff about their experiences while being treated for their physical injuries

[20]. In fact, treating nurses are the first mental health aid for many survivors with injuries [21]. Furthermore, injured survivors will often gain referrals from the hospital, the treating doctor or nurse, to mental health aid professionals, as the injuries indicate the need for perhaps psychological counselling [22]. In fact, non-terrorism studies show that injured trauma survivors with a referral of a physician will have eight times more chance to seek out mental health aid than those without such a referral [23].

### *8.2.3 Having Mental Health Issues Can Limit Access to Professional Mental Health Aid*

In general, seeking out aid is often more connected with exposure than with having PTSD. For example, the Paris-2015 attack studies show that having PTSD meant less regular treatment, while direct exposure was related to having more regular treatment [24]. In fact, half of those with PTSD received no mental health treatment [9]. Such observation are also found in studies in Norway or after 9/11 that show that the better predictor for mental health aid for survivors is exposure [25, 26].

This also holds true for parents seeking aid for their child. After 9/11, parents seeking out mental health aid for their children did this mainly because of their child's exposure to the attacks, not due to perceived PTSD [27]. Similar observations were found in parents in Norway after the Utoya attacks, where PTSD in their child did not predict visits to a general practitioner [28]. These observations follow non-disaster studies. For example, one study showed that of those with PTSD, only 10% seek out aid [29].

### *8.2.4 Stigma*

Stigma has been found to be an important barrier in seeking out mental health aid. In non-terrorism studies, stigma has been found to be a factor holding people back from seeking out aid [30, 31]. So too for terrorism studies. As one of the survivors of the Belgium attacks stated:

> *"Everybody has a right on a burn-out these days. There was someone who had to do administrative tasks, and he was suddenly gone: burn-out... And then you get your own mental problems, and you think, they're going to compare me with that guy. You're there with REAL problems, and someone else... So, yeah, psychosocial wellbeing, it has a dirty side to it"* [19].

Stigma can be deeply rooted in the culture of a country. In some cultures, experiencing mental health issues is a sign of weakness, while in others there is an openness to the topic that allows easier access to mental health aid [32].

## 8.3 Steps in Accessing Professional Mental Health Aid

For those that are able to access the professional mental health aid, there are other issues. The process to actually accessing aid can be long. Studies indicate that even if survivors find the way to aid, it might not always be that this was satisfactory or perceived as competent [7].

### *8.3.1 Recognizing the Mental Health Issues*

The survivor does not need help

The first step towards accessing mental health aid is recognizing that there is an issue that needs help [19]. This is not straightforward, however. Often people feel they do not have a problem. For example, a study after 9/11 showed that among those with mental health issues, 73% felt they did not have a problem [10]. In fact, this was more common that financial issues or problems accessing services [10]. This explains also why having mental health issues such as PTSD or depression is not always a predictor of whether or not someone will seek out professional mental health aid [17].

That is a major difference between survivors with mental health issues. Some recognize their problems quite immediately, while others deny them and learn to live with them. This would explain why, when survivors do seek out help, they tend to do it in the first year. After the first year, the chance of seeking out professional mental health aid for those with mental health disorders is a lot lower [11, 33].

– Mental health literacy

This problem recognizing mental health issues might be related to a lack of mental health literacy [19]. For example, one study after the Paris attacks showed that half of those with PTSD did not want mental health aid, whether because they felt it was not the right time for them, or because they felt no need for it [9]. Mental health itself can be an idea that seems abstract, and not part of one's daily world. For example, after 9/11, one of the hypotheses why Asian Americans sought out less aid was due to a different cultural understanding of mental health issues [11].

This is also evident in the fact that parents after both the Utoya attacks as well as after 9/11 did not seek out professional mental health aid for their child because of PTSD, but because the child had experienced the exposure to the attacks [27, 28]. Meaning that the fact of someone being present near a terrorist attack is seen as a reason to send a child to professional mental health, but less so for the actual symptoms a child might experience.

– Hitting rock bottom

However, sometimes survivor only seek out aid once they hit so-called rock-bottom. One survivor recounted *"I got guns at home, and there was screaming on the square in my village, and I thought, what's going on here? So, I took my gun and ammunition, was waiting by the door, and thought, if someone comes in here... But it was nothing. And then I said to myself: 'Maybe I should talk with a psychologist'"* [19]

Other reasons stopping survivors can be stigma or feeling that acknowledging that they have issues, means adjusting their social role. For example, a mother might feel that her having mental health issues would change her role as a mother [22].

– Social support

In this case, the social support can be both a factor that improves access, as well as one that limits it [19, 34]. The social support can showcase the mental health issues one experiences and encourage access. Furthermore, when the social support is in the form of victim support groups, it is related to continued access to mental health care [9]. However, the social support might also lead to a lack of acknowledgement of the issues. For example, other studies have found that survivors sometimes choose to handle their problems on their own, and rely on their social support [14, 16, 19]. This is quite common for all types of disasters and trauma [32, 35].

Social acknowledgement of mental health issues in society is therefore important: if the idea of mental health issues due to trauma is not widely accepted in society, or the community, it forms a natural barrier in seeking out aid [19, 32, 36]. However, equally, the social support might actually add to the idea that the person can handle the issues by themselves [19]. Indeed, as someone from a non-terrorism study states:

> "*Even today the people in my surroundings don't have the faintest idea what it means to be traumatized. They simply can't imagine it and are/were therefore not helpful.*" [32]

## 8.3.2 *Incentive to Access Aid*

Related to this recognition is taking the first step towards professional mental health aid. It indeed might be that the survivor realizes it, but cannot take the first step towards aid [19, 37]. As one survivor mentioned:

> "*'I thought long about that (going to therapy). But to do it... Then you have to take the step to be involved with that. And that's what was hard for me, to be occupied with that. Because—you get confronted again with everything. And, just, you know, if you do it, it's going to be tough, and taking the step on your own to go is already tough. So yeah, you got to do it all again on your own, you know*" [19]

A parent of a child who was killed in the Utoya attacks stated:

> "*I still feel the need to talk to someone but at the same time it is just too much effort figuring out who to contact and how (...) the help should have lasted longer (...) the most important thing is that the system for help does not let us go, because we have a very hard time asking for help and saying what kind of help we need.*" [37]

Another stated:

*"Accept help...you must be willing to accept and seek out help. After a while, nobody shows up at your door and asks you whether you need anything. You must accept and seek out help. I think that has been the most important part"* [37].

Furthermore, the step can seem even larger due to the mental health issues. For example, survivors might experience severe fear for other people [38].

In addition, a significant barrier might be the lack of knowledge of mental health services. In fact, studies seem to indicate that awareness of mental health services is quite low. One study found only 20% of people who had experienced mass violence knew of mental health services following mass violence, with roughly one in five having used any support service [39]. What seems important is prior experience with mental health services [40]. A study on people after school shootings showed that prior emotional problems predicted mental health usage [41].

General practitioners can be important in making the step. After many terrorist attacks, the general practitioner was the first contact point for any mental health issues [28, 42]. In Norway, for example, PTSD predicated a higher frequency of visits to the general practitioner [13]. Considering the importance of general practitioner in the early aftermath of an attack, it has been suggested that they need to be incorporated into crisis management plans for disasters and terrorism [43]. However, the lack of mental health literacy can also hold true for general practitioners. Non-terrorism trauma studies have shown that general practitioners can have difficulties recognizing symptoms of PTSD [44–46]. Related to this lack of knowledge is that general practitioners, despite being the first contact point, often become the last contact point; in other words, they fail to refer the survivor to adequate aid [32, 47]. A final point on this is of course this very much depends on the healthcare system as well. For example, survivors of the Paris attacks often went directly to specialized services, and used the general practitioner a lot less [24].

That would explain results from studies after Oklahoma City Bombing, that show that half of those with PTSD, while receiving mostly some form of aid, never went to a psychiatrist [33]. Similarly, while after the Paris attacks, despite suffering from at least one mental health disorder, half of those exposed never received multiple session psychological care [9].

### *8.3.3 Issues with Professional Mental Healthcare Providers*

Aside from the issues with navigating the mental healthcare system, there are issues with finding a professional that has the right expertise and the necessary understanding of the problem.

Studies from parents of deceased children after the attacks in Oslo indicated that they at times did not feel understood by the mental health professionals or felt left alone [37]. This issue was also found in Belgian studies [19]. Survivors of the attacks often felt dissatisfied with the expertise of the professionals, or simply with their lack of being able to understand what they had gone through. As one survivor stated:

> "*'[Therapists] aren't prepared for something like this. And I think there's a huge gap there, both with victim support as with psychologists, that there isn't a specialization in trauma-care. It doesn't exist...*" [19]

Survivors with PTSD will often be more dissatisfied with the aid they receive [11]. This might be because they hope for a miracle cure of their symptoms, or, it might be, because in general, people with mental health issues tend to have an affected perception of social relationships and support [14].

Additionally, while financial issues are often not a barrier in accessing the professional mental health aid, they might be barriers in continuing it. Whether in the United States, Norway, Belgium or the United Kingdom, financial aspects can form a barrier [10, 48]. For example, in Belgium, seeking aid that the survivor perceives as competent might be more expensive and not covered by insurance funds [19]. In addition, survivors often have to deal with their mental health issues while trying to still secure an income. This can lead to situations where survivors have to work less due to the professional mental health aid, while still experiencing barriers. For example, one study on United Kingdom survivors showed that a third had to reduce their working hours, and others took sick leave [42]. As one survivor stated:

> *"You have to make an estimation of the costs. Yeah, but how can you know beforehand? All those medical costs? And I think that the insurances handled that way too quickly. I mean, for us – it might not be financial problem, because we have money, but others without a doubt will have problems. Yeah... People just have to find their way on their own, which basically means the insurances want to ignore them (because the process is so complex and difficult). I just filled in the papers – they have been here for a half a year, because it was just so intimidating, like "How do I start this?""* [19]

## 8.4 Improving Professional Mental Health Aid Access

To end this chapter, the question that any public health policy makers would want answered is how to improve the access? In fact, the difficulty answering of that question in terms of public health policy is quite well known [49].

One idea is early outreach and the creation of hubs for survivors. This would solve several issues that are common in the immediate aftermath of attacks. After the 2019 Utrecht attack, half of the victims still needed aid in finding the right help [50], while studies after the Manchester attack also point to the problem of giving appropriate psychosocial care in the immediate aftermath [51]. After the Paris attacks, then again, there was a high amount of psychomedical care in the 48 h following the attacks [24, 52].

While the preparation of such outreach programs is the subject of the next chapter, it is worthwhile to see in short if these programs solve the issues described in this chapter.

### 8.4.1 Project Liberty

Project Liberty was the project set up in the aftermath of 9/11 for those who needed counseling, and was the largest program of its kind in history [53]. Project Liberty was free for people to use, thus eliminating one potential access barrier, and was widely advertised and promoted throughout New York City [54, 55]. However, other barriers persisted even, such as the lack of experience of psychologists and therapists with trauma and PTSD [54]. Despite this, 89% of those who received the services rated it as good or excellent [56].

This of course does not mean that 89% of those that used the services had in fact problems. As Chap. 5 of this book showed, resilience is quite common reaction after terrorism [57]. Furthermore, there is a risk of bias: if people with access problems have mental health issues, those that contact the services are in theory more likely be those that have no PTSD or other problems, yet the results showcase that 26% and 16% of the recipients had PTSD and depression respectively; in fact, 40% of the recipients of counseling had mental health issues [58]. In total, 9% of the recipients were referred to professional mental health services [59].

### 8.4.2 Other Outreach Programs

Similar to Project Liberty, the UK had the resilience hub after the Manchester Arena bombing. The studies on this hub show that such hubs are a good initiative, but that they are not a miracle cure. In fact, like with Project Liberty, not everyone will be happy, and not every survivor will reach it. Even when advertised, and even when free, there are access barriers that remain [51, 60].

The UK also had the Screen and Treat Programme for survivors of attacks in Tunesia, Paris, and Brussels. However, the programme was seen as being too late for survivors, despite seeing the aid as well-delivered [42].

Early outreach was also a success in Norway, where 87% of the survivors were contacted by authorities, and 73.1% eventually had contact with a professional. In fact, only 14% reported unmet needs [61].

However, while successful, these programs cannot ensure that no one has mental health issues. In fact, what the goal of these programs mainly is to provide people who might develop problems with a quick way of accessing professional mental health aid.

## 8.5 Conclusion

There are many different barriers to accessing mental health aid in survivors. On the individual level, it seems that not knowing one has mental health issues is a major barrier, as is stigma. Additionally, even when making the step to seeking out aid, finding the mental health aid that suits them is difficult. It is here that prior experience with mental health aid is an advantage.

From a public health perspective, it seems that the public health programs that were shortly described provide important lessons. While indeed, no policy will ever reach everyone, nor can (or should) policy force people to seek out aid, it seems that large scale media campaigns help, as well as free access to care immediately available after the attacks is key.

Additionally, a common problem is the lack of experience of psychologists or therapists with trauma-related mental health issues. This both hampers treatment and also pushes survivors away. In addition to access, there should be focus on ensuring that survivors keep on seeking out aid when they experience problems. What is related to this continued aid seeking is the motivation and help from victim support groups, but also, a general societal acknowledgement that indeed people might suffer from problems. One slogan in the aftermath of 9/11 was for example "Even heroes need to talk" [54]. In the aftermath of disaster, time is key, and the first year is important to ensure that survivors who need aid actually receive the aid they need.

## References

1. Neria Y, Nandi A, Galea S. Post-traumatic stress disorder following disasters: a systematic review. Psychol Med. 2008;38:467–80.
2. Slone M, Mann S. Effects of war, terrorism and armed conflict on young children: a systematic review. Child Psychiatry Hum Dev. 2016;47:950–65.
3. Paz García-Vera M, Sanz J, Gutiérrez S. A systematic review of the literature on posttraumatic stress disorder in victims of terrorist attacks. Psychol Rep. 2016;119:328–59.
4. Perlman SE, Friedman S, Galea S, et al. Short-term and medium-term health effects of 9/11. Lancet. 2011;378:925–34.
5. Rubin GJ, Wessely S. The psychological and psychiatric effects of terrorism. Psychiatr Clin N Am. 2013;36:339–50.
6. Rodriguez JJ, Kohn R. Use of mental health services among disaster survivors. Curr Opin Psychiatry. 2008;21:370–8.
7. Nordström E-EL, Kaltiala R, Kristensen P, et al. Bereaved parents' and siblings' healthcare needs, healthcare utilization, and satisfaction with healthcare services eight years after the 2011 Utøya terror attack. Death Stud. 2025;49:1363–75.
8. Strøm IF, Wentzel-Larsen T, Stensland S, et al. Health care needs, experiences, and satisfaction after terrorism: a longitudinal study of parents of survivors of the Utøya attack. BMC Health Serv Res. 2024;24:277.
9. Pirard P, Motreff Y, Stene LE, et al. Initiation of multiple-session psychological care in civilians exposed to the November 2015 Paris terrorist attacks. Arch Public Health. 2023;81:207.

10. Boscarino JA, Adams RE, Stuber J, et al. Disparities in mental health treatment following the World Trade Center Disaster: implications for mental health care and health services research. J Trauma Stress. 2005;18:287–97.
11. Jacobson MH, Norman C, Nguyen A, et al. Longitudinal determinants of depression among World Trade Center Health Registry enrollees, 14–15 years after the 9/11 attacks. J Affect Disord. 2018;229:483–90.
12. Stene LE, Thoresen S, Wentzel-Larsen T, et al. Healthcare utilization after mass trauma: a register-based study of consultations with primary care and mental health services in survivors of terrorism. BMC Psychiatry. 2022;22:720.
13. Haga JM, Thoresen S, Stene LE, et al. Healthcare to parents of young terrorism survivors: a registry-based study in Norway. BMJ Open. 2017;7:e018358.
14. Stevens GJ, Dunsmore JC, Agho KE, et al. Coping support factors among Australians affected by terrorism: 2002 Bali bombing survivors speak. Med J Aust. 2013;199:772–5.
15. Boscarino JA, Adams RE, Figley CR. Mental health service use 1-year after the World Trade Center disaster: implications for mental health care. Gen Hosp Psychiatry. 2004;26:346–58.
16. Stuber J, Galea S, Boscarino JA, et al. Was there unmet mental health need after the September 11, 2001 terrorist attacks? Soc Psychiatry Psychiatr Epidemiol. 2006;41:230–40.
17. Boscarino JA, Galea S, Ahern J, et al. Utilization of mental health services following the September 11th terrorist attacks in Manhattan, New York City. Int J Emerg Ment Health. 2002;4:143–55.
18. Fuertes JN, Mislowack A, Bennett J, et al. The physician–patient working alliance. Patient Educ Couns. 2007;66:29–36.
19. Van Overmeire R, Muysewinkel E, Van Keer R-L, et al. Victims of the terrorist attacks in Belgium and professional mental health aid barriers: a qualitative study. Front Psychiatry. 2021;12. Epub ahead of print 2 July https://doi.org/10.3389/fpsyt.2021.638272.
20. Bugge I, Jensen TK, Nilsen LG, et al. Psychosocial care for hospitalized young survivors after the terror attack on Utøya Island: a qualitative study of the survivors' experiences. Injury. 2019;50:197–204.
21. Garfield R. Commentary: the evolving role of nurses in terrorism and war. Am J Infect Control. 2003;31:163–7.
22. Van Overmeire R, Van Keer R, Bilsen J. Impact of terrorist attacks on social relationships. Clin Psychol Psychother. 2021;28:1472–81.
23. Wong EC, Schell TL, Marshall GN, et al. Mental health service utilization after physical trauma. Med Care. 2009;47:1077–83.
24. Pirard P, Baubet T, Motreff Y, et al. Use of mental health supports by civilians exposed to the November 2015 terrorist attacks in Paris. BMC Health Serv Res. 2020;20:959.
25. Stene LE, Wentzel-Larsen T, Dyb G. Healthcare needs, experiences and satisfaction after terrorism: a longitudinal study of survivors from the utøya attack. Front Psychol. 7. Epub ahead of print 24 November 2016 https://doi.org/10.3389/fpsyg.2016.01809.
26. Boscarino JA, Adams RE, Figley CR. Mental health service use after the World Trade Center Disaster. J Nerv Ment Dis. 2011;199:91–9.
27. DeVoe ER, Bannon WM, Klein TP. Post-9/11 helpseeking by New York City parents on behalf of highly exposed young children. Am J Orthopsychiatry. 2006;76:167–75.
28. Haga JM, Stene LE, Thoresen S, et al. Does posttraumatic stress predict frequency of general practitioner visits in parents of terrorism survivors? A longitudinal study. Eur J Psychotraumatol. 2017;8 https://doi.org/10.1080/20008198.2017.1389206.
29. Wang PS, Berglund P, Olfson M, et al. Failure and delay in initial treatment contact after first onset of mental disorders in the national comorbidity survey replication. Arch Gen Psychiatry. 2005;62:603.
30. Clement S, Schauman O, Graham T, et al. What is the impact of mental health-related stigma on help-seeking? A systematic review of quantitative and qualitative studies. Psychol Med. 2015;45:11–27.

31. Corrigan PW, Druss BG, Perlick DA. The impact of mental illness stigma on seeking and participating in mental health care. Psychol Sci Public Interest. 2014;15:37–70.
32. Schreiber V, Maercker A, Renneberg B. Social influences on mental health help-seeking after interpersonal traumatization: a qualitative analysis. BMC Public Health. 2010;10:634.
33. Tucker P, Pfefferbaum B, Jeon-Slaughter H, et al. Extended mental health service utilization among survivors of the Oklahoma City bombing. 2014;65:559–62.
34. Ghuman SJ, Brackbill RM, Stellman SD, et al. Unmet mental health care need 10–11 years after the 9/11 terrorist attacks: 2011–2012 results from the World Trade Center Health Registry. BMC Public Health. 2014;14:491.
35. Kantor V, Knefel M, Lueger-Schuster B. Perceived barriers and facilitators of mental health service utilization in adult trauma survivors: a systematic review. Clin Psychol Rev. 2017;52:52–68.
36. Maercker A, Müller J. Social acknowledgment as a victim or survivor: a scale to measure a recovery factor of PTSD. J Trauma Stress. 2004;17:345–51.
37. Fjærestad A, Stige SH, Dyregrov A, et al. Terror-bereaved parents experiences of professional help and support: a qualitative analysis. Eur J Psychotraumatol. 2025;16 https://doi.org/10.1080/20008066.2025.2529743.
38. Filkuková P, Hafstad GS, Jensen TK. Who can I trust? Extended fear during and after the Utøya terrorist attack. Psychol Trauma. 2016;8:512–9.
39. Rancher C, Moreland AD, Galea S, et al. Awareness and use of support services following mass violence incidents. J Psychiatr Res. 2024;180:79–85.
40. Felix ED, Janson M, Fly J. Factors affecting mental health service use among university students following an episode of mass violence. Psychol Trauma. 2021;13:263–70.
41. Reffi AN, Ellis RA, Darnell BC, et al. Mental health service utilization following a campus mass shooting: the role of preshooting emotion dysregulation and posttraumatic cognitions. Psychol Trauma. 2022;14:151–60.
42. Cyhlarova E, Knapp M, Mays N. Responding to the mental health consequences of the 2015–2016 terrorist attacks in Tunisia, Paris and Brussels: implementation and treatment experiences in the United Kingdom. J Health Serv Res Policy. 2020;25:172–80.
43. Clary B, Baert B, Bourrel G, et al. Integrating general practitioners into crisis management would accelerate the transition from victim to effective professional: qualitative analyses of a terrorist attack and catastrophic flooding. Eur J Gen Pract. 2022;28:125–33.
44. Sugg NK, Inui T. Primary care physicians' response to domestic violence. Opening Pandora's box. JAMA. 1992;267:3157–60.
45. Reid SA, Glasser M. Primary care physicians' recognition of and attitudes toward domestic violence. Acad Med. 1997;72:51–3.
46. Munro CG, Freeman CP, Law R. General practitioners' knowledge of post-traumatic stress disorder: a controlled study. Br J Gen Pract. 2004;54:843–7.
47. Frueh BC, Cousins VC, Hiers TG, et al. The need for trauma assessment and related clinical services in a state-funded mental health system. Community Ment Health J. 2002;38:351–6.
48. Stene LE, Dyb G. Health service utilization after terrorism: a longitudinal study of survivors of the 2011 Utøya attack in Norway. BMC Health Serv Res. 2015;15:158.
49. Kleber RJ. Trauma and public mental health: a focused review. Front Psychiatry. 2019;10 https://doi.org/10.3389/fpsyt.2019.00451.
50. Bosmans MWG, Plevier C, Schutz F, et al. The impact of a terrorist attack: survivors' health, functioning and need for support following the 2019 Utrecht tram shooting 6 and 18 months post-attack. Front Psychol. 2022;13 https://doi.org/10.3389/fpsyg.2022.981280.
51. Stancombe J, Williams R, Drury J, et al. People's experiences of distress and psychosocial care following a terrorist attack: interviews with survivors of the Manchester Arena bombing in 2017. BJPsych Open. 2022;8:e41.
52. Vandentorren S, Pirard P, Sanna A, et al. Healthcare provision and the psychological, somatic and social impact on people involved in the terror attacks in January 2015 in Paris: cohort study. Br J Psychiatry. 2018;212:207–14.

53. Pfefferbaum B. Disasters in the 21st century: lessons from project liberty. Psychiatr Serv. 2006;57:1251.
54. Sederer LI, Lanzara CB, Essock SM, et al. Lessons learned from the New York state mental health response to the September 11, 2001. Attacks. 2011;62:1085–9.
55. Frank RG, Pindyck T, Donahue SA, et al. Impact of a media campaign for disaster mental health counseling in post-September 11 New York. 2006;57:1304–8.
56. Jackson CT, Allen G, Essock SM, et al. Clients' satisfaction with project liberty counseling services. Psychiatr Serv. 2006;57:1316–9.
57. Bonanno GA. Loss, trauma, and human resilience: have we underestimated the human capacity to thrive after extremely aversive events? Am Psychol. 2004;59:20–8.
58. Jackson CT, Allen G, Essock SM, et al. Clusters of event reactions among recipients of project liberty mental health counseling. 2006;57:1271–6.
59. Covell NH, Essock SM, Felton CJ, et al. Characteristics of project liberty clients that predicted referrals to intensive mental health services. Psychiatr Serv. 2006;57:1313–5.
60. Stancombe J, Williams R, Drury J, et al. Trajectories of distress and recovery, secondary stressors and social cure processes in people who used the resilience hub after the Manchester Arena bombing. BJPsych Open. 2023;9:e143.
61. Dyb G, Jensen T, Glad KA, et al. Early outreach to survivors of the shootings in Norway on the 22nd of July 2011. Eur J Psychotraumatol. 2014;5 https://doi.org/10.3402/ejpt.v5.23523.

# Chapter 9
# Lessons from the Past for the Challenges of Tomorrow: Preparedness, Response, Recovery, and Psychosocial Plans for Terrorism

## 9.1 Introduction

The headline of a slightly buried article of a Belgian newspaper, published on the 5th of February 2026, read "*Minister Verlinden finally makes work of a 'unique contact point' for terror, ten years after the attacks*" [1]. Belgium is an unfortunate example of a country that, due to circumstances, had no long-term plan for "recovery," despite a quite good preparedness and response [2, 3].

Preparedness, response, and recovery are the three key words for any plan involving terrorism, or any disaster for that matter [4, 5]:

- Preparedness is everything before the attacks.
- Response is everything after the attacks, up to 4 to 6 weeks after the attacks.
- Recovery is the phase where those who are still distressed are focussed on.

However, despite how essential these concepts are, there is a surprising lack of empirical evidence for how to do this for psychosocial plans: there is no golden standard, and furthermore, what works in one country, might not work in another [6]. While there are many expert-based guidelines, they are not based on evidence, but on experience [7]. These expert experiences are certainly valuable, but again, it is unclear what value they have in terms of generalizations [2]. Furthermore, it seems that these guidelines do not translate exactly to reality; every country seems to adjust the guidelines to their own needs, or ignore certain aspects [8].

In this chapter, a summary will be made of the research available, and an attempt will be made to create a cohesive structure that provides general principles, not based on expert opinions, but on research of actual experiences in the field. Though, again, it is important to reiterate there is no gold standard [6].

The structure this chapter will follow is the structure of psychosocial planning for terrorism is divided: preparedness for attacks, response in the aftermath of attacks, and the recovery in the long-term for survivors.


R. Van Overmeire, *Terrorism, Mental Health and Aftercare*,
https://doi.org/10.1007/978-3-032-31560-1_9

## 9.2 Preparedness

Preparedness is essential for any response. A response without preparedness might lead to large caveats and issues, while preparedness with a plan helps making sense of a situation [9]. In fact, survivors, and society at large, might feel anger, feeling of unsafety and a sense of unpredictability when it becomes clear there was no structure or plan to any psychosocial aid provided [10]. As such, preparedness has a mental health purpose in itself, namely: a plan executed provides a sense of coherence and the idea that rescue workers and the government know what they are doing.

Preparedness has two elements to it. The first element is the historical preparedness, that comes to exist through previous experiences. As such, sometimes preparedness systems are adjusted because they are seen to fail in practice in the response to a disaster. For example, in the recovery phase of the terrorist attacks of Belgium, it was clear that providing long-term mental health aid for survivors was limited due to the structure of the federal state: the transfer of the mental health aid of the federal level to the regional level was limited because of the unclarity of responsibilities [2].

Clearly, this preparedness coming forth from experience is inherent to a country and is difficult to transfer to other countries, due to it often being very specific to geography, healthcare systems, etc.—after all, the complexity of the French federal state is not the same type of complexity of Belgian or Norway [2].

The second element are the principles that are true for all systems, and that are often based on common sense ideas. These are:

1. First, even in systems where disaster preparedness is high, there will still be limitations in preparedness [11]. As risk analysis teaches, there is always a risk, no matter the preparation [12].
2. Secondly, pre-event planning is important, but, paradoxically perhaps at first sight, it is also very important to have flexible models to deliver psychosocial aid [13]. The reason being that disasters are unique: there is no disaster that requires the exact same response. Neither are there terrorist attacks that are the same and require the same psychosocial approach. An attack as large as 9/11 will require a city-wide approach, as most New Yorkers were indeed affected [14], while a more local attack, such as the attack of the Jewish museum in Belgium in 2015, will require perhaps a more focussed approach.
3. Third, and related to the previous point: there is always a gap between the post-disaster plans and the actual response [7]. Effective and coordinated delivery of proper mental health aid in a post-disaster setting is a difficult task, no matter the planning [15], and a plan is a guide, not something that can be followed to the letter. Disasters can happen anywhere, and the scale, nor length, is known beforehand [9].
4. Fourth, related to the third point, is that plans need to stay up to date. They need to incorporate changes in government structures, local levels, etc., yet this aspect of preparedness is often overlooked [9].

5. Fifth, to have an efficient preparedness with regards to psychosocial care, it is a common-sense principle that the relevant disciplines (e.g. mental health sciences and behavioural sciences) need to be integrated into the general disaster planning [16, 17]. This often remains lacking in many disaster plans [18], which often lack involvement of mental health experts, such as psychiatrists [19]. In general, a multi-disciplinary approach is essential in psychosocial care after disasters [20]. It is impossible to only focus on rescue work or only focus on psychosocial care. There is a need to bring together different disciplines to ensure the best possible preparedness and response possible.
6. Finally, in any country, cooperation between agencies is important, and can be facilitated before any attack [21].

**Black Swans**

Disaster preparedness and psychosocial care after disasters need to be flexible, because it can never be predicted what form a disaster will take. As Nassim Nicholas Taleb quotes Donald Rumsfeld in Black Swan to showcase this principle: there are the known knowns, the known unknowns and the unknown unknowns [22]. Disaster preparedness can only take into account the known known and the known unknowns. For example, it needs to be known how the healthcare system works, so that the psychosocial response does not consider things that are impossible. Similarly, while one cannot know when, how, or where a disaster strikes, general principles, as highlighted in this book, can help. However, even knowing all that, there is no bulletproof system, and there will always be mistakes that become known only once the mistakes have happened.

There are several specific aspects that can be prepared with regard to disasters and terrorist attacks:

### *9.2.1 Documentation Protocol*

It is of the upmost importance to register those directly exposed to terrorist attacks, for two main reasons [9]:

1. Registration provides comfort and assurance to loved ones.
2. Registration is essential for the recovery phase.

In practice, information is often written down on paper, with incomplete information [3, 23]. One of the main lessons from the October 7 attacks in Israel is the importance of having a standardized documentation protocol for survivors [23]. Therefore, it should be decided in advance: what information is needed? [9]

A lack of proper registration seems to lead to problems in the recovery phase [9], as evident from the Belgian recovery phase, which had a surprising low amount of people contacted for psychosocial aid [24].

### 9.2.2 Traumatology

A reoccurring problem after some terrorist attacks is the lack of expertise in psychologists with experience in trauma-responses [25, 26]. It is therefore worthwhile to provide training for healthcare providers in psychological first aid (see Sect. 9.2.5.), which is an easy way of providing support in the immediate aftermath of a disaster. This can be integrated into education, or in preparation exercises [17].

### 9.2.3 Training

Training for providing mental health support, as well as knowing any psychosocial care plan, is essential for healthcare providers to know [9, 17]. As seen in studies, in the chaos of a disaster, communication and knowing each other is essential in a disaster response [3]. Furthermore, training familiarizes rescue workers with the plans [9].

However, the mental health aspects need to be integrated into the general disaster trainings, which is often not the case [17, 27], yet this is essential, as first responders are not used to providing psychosocial care in emergency settings [27]. Terrorist attacks are a very uncommon occurrence, which are also related with a lot of threat (and thus stress), especially for those on the scene of the crime [3]. Training provides a framework and gives guidelines for what is essential and reduces the risk of common mistakes in the organization of the immediate post-disaster mental health aid, such as documenting survivors or ensuring the place where first mental health aid is provided is not on the scene of the attack.

Training also provides clarity on several important factors.

1. Who leads the mental health aid in the aftermath?
2. Who does what in the aftermath? [28]

The question that is, unfortunately, difficult to answer, is who is best fit to lead the psychosocial care in the immediate aftermath, as there is little research on this aspect [29]. It cannot be assumed that a unit head or department head is best fit to lead in an emergency situation, as it cannot be underestimated how much stress can influence the judgement of experienced healthcare professionals in action [3]. Either way, disaster management in general is important, and should be an area in which investments are beneficial [9, 30]. This disaster management can also be tested during trainings.

The reason trainings are often not focussed on is due to their financial costs, and a lack of time of rescue workers [9]. Additionally, political priorities might not be aligned with the need for them, as the need for trainings is often only obvious after an attack occurs [9].

One solution might be to offer online training for experts and professionals on psychosocial care [31]. For example, one study taught nurses psychological first aid online, and showed good results in how the nurses learned psychological first aid [32]. That being said, it is naturally preferrable to train in actual in-person trainings, as aspects that might be subconscious, such as posture while providing psychological first aid, cannot be properly assessed while being taught online.

### 9.2.4 Groups

What profiles do the mental health aid groups need, and how large should these be? [23] Experience shows these should be small, to avoid burnout, and should include one professional, who is further aided by volunteers who receive a basic training in PFA and recognizing mental health issues [23, 33].

### 9.2.5 General Practitioners

Many survivors reach out to their general practitioner (GP) to discuss their mental health reactions after an attack. Considering the role of GPs in the aftermath of disasters, GPs should play a bigger role in disaster planning [34–36]. GPs are the easiest contact point for survivors, and thus, GPs should know what trauma-specific symptoms are important to take note off, and to whom they should send survivors in case of mental health issues, or how to provide psychological first aid or provide psychoeducation (see Sect. 9.3.3.) [37].

### 9.2.6 Recognize and Decrease Existing Professional Mental Health Aid Barriers

Chapter 8 showed a numerous amount of mental health barriers for survivors of terrorist attacks. Trying to remove these barriers is the best preparation possible. Solutions to these barriers are increasing mental health literacy, increasing social acknowledgement of mental health problems to reduce stigma and investing in specializations on traumatology [26, 38, 39].

## 9.3 Response

In the immediate aftermath, public health policy makers should immediately start organizing a psychosocial response. The response is important and might be the defining factor in how communities recover from terrorist attacks [10]. It matters how psychosocial care is provided, and bad experiences can act as secondary stressors for survivors [40, 41].

Time is of the essence in responding to a disaster [42], yet at the same time, it is through time that a lot of issues disappear. For example, in London, 2 weeks after the attacks, distress symptoms decreased from 40% to 50% in the population to roughly 10% after 7 months [42]. Indeed, as has been mentioned in Chaps. 2 and 5 of this book, most survivors will recover naturally or be resilient [43, 44], yet, for some, aid will be necessary, and it is essential that these are identified early on [10].

While it is difficult to assess what the best psychosocial care response is within a disaster setting [45], studies do give indicators of essential aspects for any response, that will be discussed below.

### *9.3.1 Principles of Public Health Response*

The steps in community focussed public health responses that can be followed are [28]:

1. Outreach
2. Psychoeducation/psychological first aid
3. Social support
4. Assessment and follow-up to see if distress faded or increased

In providing this psychosocial care, three principles should be followed [2]:

1. Promote natural recovery
2. Identify people at risk and provide treatment when necessary
3. Lowest level psychosocial care to begin and go for more specialized when the need occurs

Another important principle is that the time is important, and the first hours and first days are the most important [46]. This is the day that survivors are documented, they received their first information on future steps, and a good establishment of who to help is important for any long-term follow-up. That does not mean that everything needs to be established in the first days (e.g. some programs for psychosocial care were only established weeks after the attack). It does mean that any psychosocial care becomes easier if in the chaos of an attack, some order is established by documentation and providing early psychoeducation and care.

Finally, as discussed in Chap. 7, social support is one of the most important buffers against mental health issues. An issue in many approaches is that while emphasizing social support and resilience, hardly any psychological approaches focus on the community, and often focus only on the individual [47]. However, it is precisely that which a public health approach should focus on: ensure that survivors have social support. Thus, it should be ensured that families are brought together, or that the social system of which the survivor is part and would be most benefited by is identified [48, 49].

### 9.3.2 Proactive Outreach

Outreach means that survivors are contacted by a special group—whether people from a central hub, or simply in another way. The goal of proactive outreach is to screen people for any problems they might have, and if need be, refer them to the proper professional mental health, or give them the proper professional mental health [50].

A proactive outreach to groups that are known to be in danger of developing mental health issues is necessary to know healthcare needs [51]. Time and again, it is clear that it is ineffective to wait for survivors with mental health issues to seek out aid on their own [42], and it is ineffective to wait for the healthcare system to go to survivors, as it is known that in the long-term, healthcare systems generally fail in responding to survivors' needs [50].

Such outreach can be quite successful in Norway, with 87% of the survivors being contacted by authorities, and 73.1% having contact with professional mental health aid. Only 14% reported unmet mental health needs [52]. It seems the groups that were the most difficult to reach were migrant families [51]. Additionally, the outreach was also successful after the 2005 London attack, leading to a high improvement for many survivors [50, 53].

However, there were variations across the country, which indicates that governmental and organizational elements play a large role in outreach [54]. For example, municipalities had a much higher success in reaching survivors than in Oslo [54]. Furthermore, in general, even with a proactive outreach, the general hinder in any outreach is the natural withdrawal of survivors [10]. It also appears that especially men might be more inclined to refuse aid [55].

Finally, to come back to the point of the importance of registering survivors: without proper registration, any outreach is doomed to fail, since it is unknown who the survivors are [24]. After the Belgian attacks, the majority of survivors who were contacted were reached within a month, but only roughly 60% of those on the registry list were contacted overall, indicating both a lack of resources, in registration lists, and in how survivors are contacted [24].

**The Norwegian Response After the Terrorist Attacks [2]**

The Norwegian case had to deal with two areas: an attack on a governmental building, and an attack on Utøya island.

The Norwegian response, like many other responses, started from Hobfoll's principles of psychological first aid: sense of safety, calming, sense of self- and community efficacy, connectedness, hope [56].

In general, acute psychosocial care was provided on municipal level by multidisciplinary teams, and was provided to victims (e.g. wounded), relatives, survivors, families and bereaved.

For the employees, a nearby hotel was used to provide psychosocial care. This is similar to the attacks in Belgium, where a hotel near the metro was also used as area to provide psychosocial care [2, 24]. Employees received the acute psychosocial care, and also received information meetings, where they received practical information.

For the children of Utoya island, a hotel nearby the island was used.

Seven hours after the attacks, a more focussed psychosocial care was organized. Relatives of injured and deceased people were helped in separate crisis centres.

In the medium-long term, watchful waiting was employed, which means that no treatment is offered until 4 weeks have passed. Additionally, the principle of lowest level of care was employed: specialized treatment was only provided when the symptom treatment required it. In short, it is a principle of proportionately.

When needed, survivors were referred to specialized treatment by regular GP. The two main treatments used were Trauma-focused Cognitive Behavioural Therapy (TF-CBT) or Eye Movement Desensitization Reprocessing (EMDR) when post-traumatic stress disorder (PTSD) was present.

Employees were helped by occupational health services, and encouraged to return to work as soon as possible, so that the employee social support and community could help recover. As Chap. 7 showed, structural social support of fellow survivors helps in the long-term.

Survivors of the Utøya were provided a designated contact person in the municipality that would help with the follow-up, practical advice, and support.

### *9.3.3 Psychosocial Support*

How to reduce distress during a disaster? In general, what most survivors will need is quite practical; in fact, most survivors will simply want information: what area is hit, how bad is the attack, etc [42, 57]. Uncertainty is avoidable. It is important to find out and address the basic needs of the community affected [42, 57]. As such, the principles of early psychosocial support are to provide protection and security and satisfy the current needs of survivors, while trying to active the social support network of survivors [58].

In the immediate aftermath of the attack, this psychosocial support should be provided away from the scene of the crime. Additionally, injured people do not need psychosocial support at that moment, and should be treated for their physical injuries; in fact, nurses often act as psychosocial support during the recovery of injured survivors [10, 59].

There are several ways of providing early psychosocial support for survivors.

- *Psychological First Aid*

Psychological first aid (PFA) is essential in the immediate response [10]. It is based on the idea that people have the strength to recover on their own, but that they just need support [60]. It is also useful in the response since it can be easily taught to lay people [56, 61]. For example, in the aftermath of the October 7 attacks in Israel, volunteers were trained to provide PFA [23], while after 9/11, many early services were mainly focussed on PFA [62].

PFA might seem complex, judging by its name, but is actually quite straightforward. It is generally provided up to 7 days after the attack [60], and involves simply listening to and comforting survivors, while providing them help to rely on their social support network (which Chap. 7 of this book has shown to be the best buffer against PTSD), while also giving information and practical support that address the needs of the survivors at that moment [63].

While overall, evidence for the quality of PFA is somewhat varying [60]. It seems to be mainly good to reduce anxiety and improve functioning, but seems to be less effective in reducing future depression or PTSD [64].

It has also been suggested that artificial intelligence might be useful in providing PFA [65]. However, the issue with this suggestion is threefold: one, reliability (e.g. hallucinations of A.I.), two, the choice of A.I. (e.g. some models are better than others), and three, in a disaster setting, applying A.I. might be quite difficult.

**Avoiding Overload**

An attack can be affecting many different communities across the country.

One approach used after the October 7 attacks in Israel was the division of the country into different zones, to ensure that survivors in all areas would receive the necessary mental health aid [23].

The choice to divide or not to divide will depend on three factors [48]:

1. Who are the survivors? (e.g. children, employees, adults, migrants…)
2. Do they all belong to the same social system? (e.g. are all survivors from the same municipality? Are the deceased from all over the country?)
3. What is the location of the attack? (e.g. is one area hit or not?)

For example, after a 1989 air crash in Norway, almost all victims were from the same company. As such, the psychosocial care was provided in that company context [48].

- *Psychoeducation*

Psychoeducation seems to be useful in making symptoms that survivors might experience seem less frightening and portrays these reactions as normal. Furthermore, psychoeducation also provides early information on seeking professional help, and even seems to lead to seeking out help easier—thus, reducing the access barriers mentioned in the previous chapter [58].

Studies have shown that psychological education might not be worse than PFA in terms of reducing mental health outcomes, though PFA remains useful in comforting and reducing the initial anxiety [66, 67].

Important in a public health approach is also to make communities aware of mental health services, since they often will not know or not reach out themselves [28]. Furthermore, this (hopefully) counteracts the access barriers that might come to be due to stigma, a lack of social acknowledgement and an overreliance on social support [26, 68].

- *Psychological Debriefings*

A psychological debriefing (sometimes appearing under the name "Critical Stress Incident Debriefing") is an early psychological intervention in the immediate aftermath of, or up to a few days after, terrorist attacks that aim to let survivors or rescue workers relive their experiences during the attacks [69–73].

There is no evidence for the usefulness of psychological debriefings—in fact, they are more likely to be harmful than not, and should be avoided at all costs [69, 72–74]. This needs to be repeated again and again, since debriefings are still either recommended or performed in the aftermath of disasters [3, 69].

**Differences Between Countries**

One study on psychosocial care in France, Belgium, and Norway showcased the large differences between the response after terrorist attacks in these three countries. They differed in their definition of "victim" (and even the use of the word), how long they followed up survivors, and even how they follow-up on them [2].

These differences can be due to geography, history, the state structure, or other factors. For example, Norway relies more on municipalities, due to geographical distances, while France has a much more centralized approach, while Belgium's approach is in the acute phase centralized, and decentralized for the recovery phase [2, 8].

An obvious observation about the response in a country is that it will depend on what is available [75]. Thus, as has been already stated: there is no golden standard.

**Manchester Attack: Relatives of Victims**
Hospitals after the Manchester attacks used the so-called Swan bereavement model. Relatives of victims were directly supported by a psychosocial support team for the first 72 h, after which they were assigned a bereavement nurse, and access to the 24/7 dedicated helpline [49].

### 9.3.4 *Assessment and Follow-Up to See If Distress Faded or Increased*

#### 9.3.4.1 Screening

Screening is the act of assessing the distress levels of survivors (see Chap. 1). Key of this is, of course, to detect and identify those that are at risk of developing long-term mental health issues [10]. Naturally, it is difficult to predict who will develop long-term mental health issues, but factors already mentioned in previous chapters should be focussed on, in addition to screening of mental health symptoms [42, 76]:

- Being directly exposed.
- Previous traumatization [77].
  - This is difficult to assess, but is very important, as there is a good chance that those develop problems due to exposure to terrorism already had issues before the trauma exposure [77, 78].
- Background factors related to higher risk for PTSD or depression.
  - Low social support.
  - Being a minority.
  - Women have a higher risk to develop PTSD.
  - Having a lower income.

However, even in this group, not everyone develops problems [42] or develops them later on. Thus, when screening, two important questions play a role [2]:

- Who will be monitored?
- For how long? (e.g. how many times will they be screened for mental health issues?)

While it should be noted that any screening methodology has limitations in terms of assessing the needs of survivors [25], screening can be very effective in identifying those who are most at risk of developing problems in the future.

Screening is done either through screen-and-treat (e.g. after positive screening, immediate care) or through screen-and-refer approaches (e.g. after positive screening, referral to appropriate care) [58].

After the Manchester attacks in the UK, the National Health Service Manchester Resilience Hub invited concert attendees to complete online screenings. They screened on stress, anxiety, mood, and functioning. This was the repeated at 3-month intervals for year, then 6-month intervals, and then after 3 years, annually. When screenings showed mental health issues, psychosocial care pathways were suggested to the survivor [40]. There is evidence that those who registered for the resilience hub early had fewer issues, and more improvements, that those who registered later. Naturally, that might also have to do with survivors who have more distress registering later, and because they have more distress, perhaps also experiencing less improvements. Either way, while weak evidence, it does indicate that such a hub is a worthwhile effort—as such, it will be discussed later more in-depth [79].

#### 9.3.4.2 Timing

While the Manchester attacks hub screened every 3 months the first year, after the attacks in Norway, the government employees were screened 3 to 4 weeks after the attacks, followed by 3–4 months, and finally 12 months later. The Utøya survivors were screened 5–6 weeks, 3 months and 1 year after the attack [2]. After the London attacks, the first screening survey was launched 2 weeks after the attacks [42].

#### 9.3.4.3 Methodology of Screening

There are several ways to screen. After the 2005 London bombing, screening was done with the International Trauma Questionnaire [50]. Those that screen positive for further treatment were provided two different types of therapy. This could be trauma-focussed cognitive-behaviour therapy (TF-CBT) or eye movement desensitization and reprocessing (EMDR) [50]. The results of this approach were better than most randomized clinical trials in terms of improvement [50].

After the Manchester attacks, the Trauma Screening Questionnaire was used, in addition to the General Anxiety Disorder-7, the Patient Health Questionnaire, and the Work and Social Adjustment Scale [33]. For children and younger people, scales used were the Children's Impact of Event scale, and subscales of the Revised Children's Anxiety and Depression Scale [33].

#### 9.3.4.4 Follow-Up

It should never be the principle to provide psychological interventions (e.g. long-term therapy) as a matter of principle for survivors. In fact, generally, it is recommended to wait the first 4 weeks after a traumatic event (the so-called watchful waiting) and have follow-up contact with the survivor within a month [58]. Thus, while assessment can happen quite soon, it should not be seen as evidence of immediate PTSD reactions. For example, a non-disaster example: after sexual assault, the distress levels measured through PTSD-scales of sexual assault survivors are up to 90% and higher. These go down to below 50% after 2–3 months [80, 81].

**Case Study: Project Liberty**
Project Liberty was the large-scale mental health aid program in the aftermath of 9/11. It was a cooperation of different mental health aid organizations, meant to streamline the aid delivery.

Demographics of those who accessed the Project Liberty services show that in the first wave it was mainly citizens of New York City (89%) [25]. After this, it became mainly those with high exposure [ 82] and those who lost family in the attacks [ 83] who received further services. Of those who received counselling, 20% were children [25]. Project Liberty provided face-to-face counselling and education, as well as outreach services (e.g. going to survivors) to around 1.2 million people in the disaster area. Half were served with just psychoeducation, the other with group or individual counselling [84].

In total, 9% of the users of Project Liberty were referred to specialized services [82].

### *9.3.5 A Centralized Hub*

One possible approach to having a unified psychosocial care approach is a central hub. A central hub can be a network of existing places (e.g. it can be a collection of healthcare providers unified under one name for clarity) or be an actual place where survivors can go. The consideration for what the hub would be is based on the terrorist attacks.

In general, it seems that hubs, such as Project Liberty after 9/11 and the Resilience Hub after the Manchester attacks, were mainly places for coordination and networking, and not physical places [41, 84]. Not having a physical place has the advantage that it can be set up a lot quicker.

Reasons for having a hub are numerous.

- First, it is important to have one centralized entry point for survivors to seek out counseling and mental health aid [87]. A common irritation for survivors of terrorism to constantly provide the same information to a fragmented victim support. Centralizing the entry point avoids unnecessary secondary traumatization, and improves mental health aid access by reducing the administrative burden [26, 40, 88].
- Second, and related to point one, the hub can also act as a central communication point for questions of people in relation to the attacks (e.g. practical questions, or questions about mental health care), which is useful in reducing barriers and stigma [42]. Indeed, a common problem in the long-term is that many survivors have not found help. For example, months after the 2019 Utrecht attack, half of

the survivors still needed aid in finding the right help [89], while studies after the Manchester attacks also point to the same issue [40, 90].

- Third, while it might seem that healthcare resources going to terrorism survivors might disrupt normal services, there is no evidence this happens [91].

Several considerations of such a hub:

- Accessibility is important. Not only should the hub be free [25], but it is important that everyone should be able to access it. For example, deaf and blind people as well [92].
- Time is important: it needs to be established quite fast [93]. A warning is therefore fit here: it is clear from UK survivors that bureaucracy can cause significant delays in the establishment of such a central hub [94].
- A hub is a sort of specialized approach to psychosocial care; it also means that the transfer of responsibilities of normal care to this hub need to be handled delicately. For example, Project Heartland after the Oklahoma City Bombing suffered from some healthcare providers not wanting to give away "agency" to the project [95]. It is why such a hub needs governmental backing [95].

A hub is certainly not a miracle cure, but for many it provides some form of help for their distress and to fast-track their access to proper aid [40]. Such hubs should be open a long time, because people might only require help later on, as seen in Project liberty [96].

**Case Study Manchester 2017 Attacks**

The Manchester 2017 attacks showcase a typical example of response, and recovery, that is very similar to other countries [25, 85].

The attacks in Manchester in 2017 consisted of a suicide bomber exploding a device during a concert, killing 22 people [86]. There was no preparedness phase, but there were response and recovery phases.

In the aftermath, a Manchester Resilience Hub was set up, which employed screen-and-refer models, stepped-care approach model (e.g. most non-interventional methods, and "stepping up" to more specific forms of mental health aid when need appears to be higher), and tailored treatment pathways (e.g. not everyone needs the same help at the same time) [33].

The response and recovery phases had three aspects: (1), a universal approach: message to anyone vicariously traumatized; (2), targeted approach: approach those directly affected; (3), phased approach: use of different communication and treatment needs across different phases [33].

Screening was done online, and invitations were sent out again every 3 months [33].

Adults at low risk were given normalizations messages and advice.

Adults with moderate stress were encouraged to go to a local service to provide brief psychological interventions.

(continued)

(continued)

Adults with high levels of stress were contacted by telephone and referred to adult mental health services [33].

The team of the hub consisted of:

- Recovery workers, who received brief training around trauma.
- Senior clinicians, who are psychologists or therapists who are trained in CBT or EMDR.

Dangers in setting up a Hub:

- In immediate aftermath, all expertise and specialization will be divided geographically. Aim is to bring them together as soon as possible [33].
- Professional and structural barriers to cooperation.
- Conflicting values (e.g. some are focussed on criminal investigation, others on different aspects).
- Need for coordination—else there is a danger of duplication and fragmentation.
- Need for centralization as soon as possible, as else the effectiveness will be limited [33].

How to prepare for building a Hub?

- Existing collaborations are important—which can exist through prior trainings.
- Similarly, trust building can happen through trainings.
- Need for a disaster management leader [33].

**Proactive Outreach or a Hub?**

Proactive outreach and a hub often go hand in hand. The big difference of a proactive outreach compared to the Hub-approach is that a proactive outreach allows the healthcare system to run as before, as survivors are reached directly. A hub is a specialized approach that is using outreach, but also allows survivors to come to the services.

Norway seemed to have employed a mainly proactive outreach (probably due to large geographical difference in where survivors lived) [2], while a hub was used after Oklahoma City Bombing (Project Heartland), 9/11 (Project Liberty), the Manchester attacks (The Resilience Hub) [41, 53, 76, 84].

However, Project Heartland shows how a hub can be combined with outreach. Staff visited all homes within a mile radius of the attack, and visited homes of survivors, victim's families, and rescue workers. Additionally, they even attended meetings and reunions of survivors [95].

In other words, this dichotomy is not absolute, and only serves to illustrate the choices disaster response can take into account.

### 9.3.6 Media Campaign

The role of a media campaign is to spread the information about professional mental health aid to the population, and especially the population affected, and convince them to seek out aid. In the aftermath of 9/11, the media campaign was able to reach mainly people in New York, where Project Liberty was mainly located [97]. After the Manchester attacks in 2017, social media and the news was used, but also mails to the ticket holders [33]. Additionally, media campaigns can service as public education on mental health, and attempt to reduce stigma [9]. For example, one campaign slogan after 9/11 was "Even Heroes Need To Talk" [25].

**Finding Survivors**

After the London 2005 attacks, a Government-funded centre was set up using emergency planning legislation to provide information, advice and counselling for survivors, while lists of names of survivors were provided by hospitals treating them. Finally, a 24-h telephone-based consultation service provided medical advice to the general population, but could also be used to refer survivors to screenings and professional help [53].

### 9.3.7 Financial Aspects

Part of the response is the aspect of financing a hub or proactive outreach. Project Liberty, after 9/11, was the largest federal disaster mental health program in the United States' history and costed more than 137 million dollars to serve around 1.5 million people [76]. However, even though it was an incredible investment, there were limitation in terms of how providers should pay their staff and services [25]. Additionally, policy makers should decide how long they wish to fund a hub, as well as how the funds should flow, and what is exactly being funded: is it the first screening alone, or also the further follow-up? [ 25]

If not for the hub, for all aspects of the psychosocial response it is important to consider *how long* it will be funded, and *what* will be funded.

### 9.3.8 Contact Person

Another approach is to provide survivors with a contact person. For example, after the Norway attacks, survivors had a contact person, who helped them with practical information, support and also ensure that screening and assessment of symptoms was continued [2]. When the contact person was not a health practitioner, they would ensure that the screenings were performed by a professional [2].

In the initial first months, having a contact person was associated with lower mental health symptoms, and be more satisfied with the help [98]. That being said, it seems a contact person's usefulness is not completely clear, though it does seem to be a good way for survivors without economic means to access healthcare, and it also serves as social support for survivors [98]. The duration of the commitment with a contact person of course depends on both parties, though in Norway, a fifth still had contact with their contact person even 2 years after the attack [98].

## 9.4 Recovery

### *9.4.1 Therapy After Positive Screening*

If survivors screen positive for certain types of distress, they can be referred to more specialized aid. Overall, there are two types of therapies that have been most recommended and used in the aftermath of terrorism:

1. Eye movement desensitization and reprocessing-therapy (EMDR)
2. Cognitive Behavioural Therapy (CBT)

Especially CBT has been most recommended as treatment for those with PTSD in the aftermath of terrorism and has been shown to be effective in both injured and non-injured survivors [27, 99, 100]. For example, after 9/11, adults with mental health issues received CBT, as well as grief interventions with attention for terrorism-related problems (e.g. information about natural grieving processes), were used [25, 101].

In the aftermath of the London attacks then again, more than 80% of survivors with PTSD received CBT [42]. However, 10% received EMDR, or a combination of EMDR and CBT [42]. CBT can also be used in non-Western contexts. For example, a CBT trial on terrorism survivors in Thailand, where the threat of terrorism was constant, showed clear improvements compared to usual care [102].

Such aid is often time limited [25, 85]. After 9/11, 10 to 12 sessions were provided [25], while a community response in the form of cognitive therapy after a car bombing in 1998 in Northern Ireland showed stark improvements with only 8 sessions [103].

**Services for Children**

Children are a special group for treatment, since they are unable to seek out aid on their own, and are therefore often dependent on their parents [2].

After Project Liberty, children of 5 to 12 years of age were treated using the Child and Parent Trauma-Focused Cognitive-Behavioural Therapy Treatment Manual [25], while for adolescents (13–21 years), the Trauma/

(continued)

(continued)

Grief-Focused Group Psychotherapy Program was employed [25]. Both of these approaches include psychoeducation, affect regulation, relaxation training, cognitive restructuring, and gradual exposure techniques [25].

In addition, school-based interventions might be useful as a form of community response, where children who survived an attack receive psychological aid, but also can rely on social support of classmates and the school system [104–106]. Schools are especially useful for the long-term follow-up, and the reintegration of children into everyday life [2].

Finally, in addition to individual therapy, family therapy might be used to employ the familial social support [107].

### *9.4.2 Return to Normal Services*

Any psychosocial response will be limited in time. For example, Project Liberty was implemented in two phases: the emergency Immediate Services Program from September 12, 2001, to June 12, 2002, and the nonemergency Regular Services Program from June 15, 2002, until December 31, 2004 [25].

The use of volunteers is also limited in time. In Israel, volunteers were only required to help in the mental health aid delivery for 2 months, before the return to normal professional services [23].

As mentioned earlier, it is important to decide how long any psychosocial response will last, and will need to balance the fact that people might only seek out or need mental health aid later on, with the consideration that there is a need to return to normal services eventually [108]. This will of course depend on the nature of the terrorist attack and the number of survivors.

### *9.4.3 Use of Other Organizations*

Some government organizations provide help based on categorizations; so, some who need help, do not receive it [109]. This creates distance towards the policy. Additionally, sometimes the governmental aid is badly organized, or is perceived to be inadequate or lacking in specific trauma-focussed expertise [26, 109]. In the path of recovery, non-governmental organizations (NGOs) can be used, and might therefore sometimes be preferred. NGOs are often freer to tailor aid to the needs of survivors, and sometimes have employees who have experienced mass traumatic events themselves [109]. For example, in the aftermath of 9/11, local NGOs were part of Project Liberty [84].

### 9.4.4 *Memorials, Memory, and Survivor Groups*

In the long term, memorial services can be organized. Such reunions, memorials, and groups are ideal for outreach to survivors that might suffer from mental health problems, but have not been able to seek out professional mental health aid [95]. This can help survivors and bereaved people with their recovery, as well as developing structural social support for survivors. For example, after the Norway attacks, reunions were organized, so that survivors and bereaved still had a chance to come together to grieve [110]. Similarly, after the Belgian attacks, memorial services were organized [111].

## 9.5 Research After Disaster

A small but essential part of the post-disaster outreach, and preparedness, is research [112]. Research on disaster response and recovery is essential to improve the preparedness in a country, but also to create more empirical basis for principles to organize psychosocial care after disasters. For example, almost 40% of the registered survivors of the attacks in Belgium were meant to be contacted, but it remains unclear why they were not [24].

Such research often is difficult to set up. It requires community engagement; there is need for trust building, mitigating concerns, ensuring that re-traumatization is avoided, and above all, showcasing that the research will have value for the survivors [113].

Furthermore, there are limitations in such research, and especially in its generalization for other disasters. For example, survivors are often lost in follow-up (e.g. survivors who are resilient will probably be less inclined to spend time on providing research data), meaning that data becomes biased and focused on just a specific subgroup of survivors [114]. Additionally, all terrorist attacks are different. The lessons from one are difficult to apply to another setting [115].

Yet, such research can be an incredible added value to general principles of disaster planning, response and recovery [116]. Such research can also add to the understanding of structural barriers, organizational issues, and other aspects relevant for terrorist attacks, but also for all attacks. There are many studies showcasing that X% of survivors have PTSD; there are relatively few indicating why these people find no help, what barriers they encounter, and what can be improved. In this way, research can add to the evaluation of the response and recovery phase, and add to the improvement of the preparedness phase [29].

## 9.6 Eight Lessons About Psychosocial Care

As summary of this chapter, one study provided a list of lessons on psychosocial care after mass traumatic events such as terrorist attacks [117]:

1. Tailor the psychosocial response to the specific disaster
2. Provide a multi-dimensional psychosocial care
3. Target at-risk population groups
4. Proactively address barriers in access to care
5. Recognise the social dimensions and sources of resilience
6. Extend the roles for mental health professionals
7. Efficiently coordinate and integrate disaster response services
8. Integrate research and evaluation into disaster response planning

## 9.7 Reflections

This chapter provided some avenues for preparedness, response and recovery. There are several elements that can be highlighted.

First, in the preparedness phase, attention for integration of mental health services seems the most pressing. Additionally, documentation protocol is essential for any success of the response and recovery phase.

Secondly, in the response phase, what is priority is the outreach to survivors, whether through a Hub or proactive outreach. In fact, all these methods can be used, of course. One can set up a Hub, have proactive outreach, and even provide survivors with a contact person.

Many elements will depend on the resources available. For example, after the major chemical disaster in India, the Bhopal disaster (discussed in Chap. 6), there simply were not enough mental health specialists available [118]. As such, some countries might not have a fully developed "Victim Support" service, or might have services more focussed on physical injuries, and less developed mental health services. Related to this is that trauma expertise will vary from country to country, even among Western countries [26, 119]. For example, in the aftermath of the Belgian attacks, it was noted by a commission that there was too little specialization in the treatment of psychological trauma, nor was it offered as a specific discipline [26].

To end, what should be avoided most of all, is the secondary traumatization by bad experiences with mental health outreach and response of the government [40]. One is reminded of what Tolstoi wrote in Resurrection: "*All these people were evidently invulnerable by and impermeable to the simplest feeling of compassion only because they held offices*" [120]. Indeed, it does seem that institutional distrust and distress are related: the more distressed someone is, the less one trusts the institutions [121].

Showcasing planning, effort, and care is not just a public health responsibility, it is also a societal responsibility, to show when a nation is attacked, the nation takes responsibility to take care of those affected. Or as the first sentence of a British report on terrorism survivors states: "*Counter-terrorism is not just about the powers we have to stop those that want to cause harm, it is also about the Government's duty to support those that are impacted by terrorism*" [122].

## References


1. Struys B. Minister Verlinden maakt eindelijk werk van 'uniek contactpunt' voor terreur, tien jaar na aanslagen. De Morgen. 2026;
2. Stene LE, Vuillermoz C, Overmeire R Van, et al. Psychosocial care responses to terrorist attacks: a country case study of Norway, France and Belgium. BMC Health Serv Res 2022; 22: 390.
3. Muysewinkel E, Vesentini L, Van Deynse H, et al. A day in the life: psychological impact on emergency responders during the 22 March 2016 terrorist attacks. Front Psychiatry. 15. Epub ahead of print 12 February 2024 https://doi.org/10.3389/fpsyt.2024.1353130.
4. Williams R, Kemp V, Burgess J, et al. Practical psychosocial care for providers of pre-hospital care: a summary of the report 'valuing staff, valuing patients'. Scand J Trauma Resusc Emerg Med. 2023;31:77.
5. Williams R, Bisson JI, Kemp V, et al. Health care planning for community disaster care. In: Textbook of disaster psychiatry. Cambridge: Cambridge University Press; 2017.
6. Stene LE, Fernandez A, Gindt M, et al.. Editorial:Recovering after terrorist attacks, large-scale accidents and other disasters: Psychosocial care responses across countries. Front Psychol. 2023;14 https://doi.org/10.3389/fpsyg.2023.1168679.
7. Te Brake H, Dückers M. Early psychosocial interventions after disasters, terrorism and other shocking events: is there a gap between norms and practice in Europe? Eur J Psychotraumatol. 2013;4 https://doi.org/10.3402/ejpt.v4i0.19093.
8. Nilsen LG, Stene LE. Preparing for the unexpected: a comparative study of policies addressing post-terror health reactions in Norway and France. Int J Ment Health Syst. 2023;17:13.
9. Jacobs J, Oosterbeek M, Tummers LG, et al. The organization of post-disaster psychosocial support in The Netherlands: a meta-synthesis. Eur J Psychotraumatol. 2019;10 https://doi.org/10.1080/20008198.2018.1544024.
10. Ursano RJ, Fullerton CS, Weisaeth L, et al. Textbook of disaster psychiatry. Cambridge; 2017.
11. Jørgensen JJ, Monrad-Hansen PW, Gaarder C, et al. Disaster preparedness should represent an augmentation of the everyday trauma system, but are we prepared? Trauma Surg Acute Care Open. 2021;6:e000760.
12. Ezell BC, Bennett SP, Von Winterfeldt D, et al. Probabilistic risk analysis and terrorism risk. Risk Anal. 2010;30:575–89.
13. World Health Organization. *Building back better: sustainable mental health car after emergencies*. 2013.
14. Covell NH, Essock SM, Felton CJ, et al. Characteristics of project liberty clients that predicted referrals to intensive mental health services. Psychiatry. 2006;57:1313–5.
15. Goldmann E, Galea S. Mental health consequences of disasters. Annu Rev Public Health. 2014;35:169–83.
16. Ruzek JI, Young BH, Cordova MJ, et al. Integration of disaster mental health services with emergency medicine. Prehosp Disaster Med. 2004;19:46–53.
17. Pfefferbaum B, Flynn BW, Schonfeld D, et al. The integration of mental and behavioral health into disaster preparedness, response, and recovery. Disaster Med Public Health Prep. 2012;6:60–6.

18. Robertson M, Pfefferbaum B, Codispoti CR, et al. Integrating authorities and disciplines into the preparedness-planning process: a study of mental health, public health, and emergency management. Am J Disaster Med. 2007;2:133–42.
19. Holmes A. System issues for psychiatrists responding to disasters. Psychiatr Clin N Am. 2004;27:541–58.
20. Gabbe BJ, Veitch W, Mather A, et al. Review of the requirements for effective mass casualty preparedness for trauma systems. A disaster waiting to happen? Br J Anaesth. 2022;128:e158–67.
21. Ranse J, Gray L, Mortelmans L, et al. Spontaneous and unplanned mass gathering events: a scoping review of health considerations for riots, civil unrest, and protest. Disaster Med Public Health Prep. 2025;19:e269.
22. Taleb NNicholas. The black swan: the impact of the highly improbable. Random House; 2016.
23. Yaniv-Rosenfeld A, Ganor O, Gaon A, et al. Providing emergency mental health support to Israeli civilians evacuated from their homes following the events of October 7th, 2023. Isr J Health Policy Res. 2025;14:39.
24. Muysewinkel E, Vesentini L, Van Deynse H, et al. The psychosocial aid response after the 22/03/2016 attacks in Belgium: a community case study. Front Public Health. 2024;12 https://doi.org/10.3389/fpubh.2024.1362021.
25. Sederer LI, Lanzara CB, Essock SM, et al. Lessons learned from the New York state mental health response to the September 11, 2001, Attacks 2011; 62:1085–1089
26. Van Overmeire R, Muysewinkel E, Van Keer R-L, et al. Victims of the terrorist attacks in Belgium and professional mental health aid barriers: a qualitative study. Front Psychiatry. 2021;12 https://doi.org/10.3389/fpsyt.2021.638272.
27. Ruzek JI, Walser RD, Naugle AE, et al. Cognitive-behavioral psychology: implications for disaster and terrorism response. Prehosp Disaster Med. 2008;23:397–410.
28. Gard BA, Ruzek JI. Community mental health response to crisis. J Clin Psychol. 2006;62:1029–41.
29. Dückers MLA, Yzermans CJ, Jong W, et al. Psychosocial crisis management: the unexplored intersection of crisis leadership and psychosocial support. Risk Hazards Crisis Public Policy. 2017;8:94–112.
30. Boin A, Bynander F. Explaining success and failure in crisis coordination. Geogr Ann Ser A Phys Geogr. 2015;97:123–35.
31. Askenazy F, Fernandez A, Altan L, et al. Remote training as a common tool for the different professionals involved in the acute phase after terror attacks across Europe: perspectives from an expert panel. Front Psychiatry. 2022;13 https://doi.org/10.3389/fpsyt.2022.915929.
32. Choi E-J, Choi Y-J. Development and effect of an interactive simulated education program for psychological first aid: a randomized controlled trial. J Nurs Manag. 2024, 2024; https://doi.org/10.1155/2024/8806047.
33. Hind D, Allsopp K, Chitsabesan P, et al. The psychosocial response to a terrorist attack at Manchester Arena, 2017: a process evaluation. BMC Psychol. 2021;9:22.
34. Burns P, Douglas K, Hu W, et al. General practitioners in the field: a qualitative study of general practitioners' experiences in disaster healthcare. Aust J Gen Pract. 2020;49:132–8.
35. Burns PL, FitzGerald GJ, Hu WC, et al. General practitioners' roles in disaster health management: perspectives of disaster managers. Prehosp Disaster Med. 2022;37:124–31.
36. Clary B, Baert B, Bourrel G, et al. Integrating general practitioners into crisis management would accelerate the transition from victim to effective professional: qualitative analyses of a terrorist attack and catastrophic flooding. Eur J Gen Pract. 2022;28:125–33.
37. Haga JM, Stene LE, Thoresen S, et al. Does posttraumatic stress predict frequency of general practitioner visits in parents of terrorism survivors? A longitudinal study. Eur J Psychotraumatol. 2017;8 https://doi.org/10.1080/20008198.2017.1389206.
38. Thoresen S, Jensen TK, Wentzel-Larsen T, et al. Social support barriers and mental health in terrorist attack survivors. J Affect Disord. 2014;156:187–93.

39. Corrigan PW, Druss BG, Perlick DA. The impact of mental illness stigma on seeking and participating in mental health care. Psychol Sci Public Interest. 2014;15:37–70.
40. Stancombe J, Williams R, Drury J, et al. People's experiences of distress and psychosocial care following a terrorist attack: interviews with survivors of the Manchester Arena bombing in 2017. BJPsych Open. 2022;8:e41.
41. Stancombe J, Williams R, Drury J, et al. Trajectories of distress and recovery, secondary stressors and social cure processes in people who used the resilience hub after the Manchester Arena bombing. BJPsych Open. 2023;9:e143.
42. Rubin GJ, Wessely S. The psychological and psychiatric effects of terrorism. Psychiatr Clin N Am. 2013;36:339–50.
43. Bonanno GA. Loss, trauma, and human resilience: have we underestimated the human capacity to thrive after extremely aversive events? Am Psychol. 2004;59:20–8.
44. Bonanno GA. The resilience paradox. Eur J Psychotraumatol. 2021;12 https://doi.org/10.1080/20008198.2021.1942642.
45. O'Neill PA. The ABC'S of disaster response. Scand J Surg. 2005;94:259–66.
46. Allsopp K, Brewin CR, Barrett A, et al. Responding to mental health needs after terror attacks. BMJ. 2019:l4828.
47. Friedman-Peleg K, Goodman YC. From posttrauma intervention to immunization of the social body: pragmatics and politics of a resilience program in Israel's periphery. Cult Med Psychiatry. 2010;34:421–42.
48. Weisæth L. Psychosocial intervention models and outcomes after a terror disaster. CNS Spectr. 2021;26:92–100.
49. Craigie RJ, Farrelly PJ, Santos R, et al. Manchester Arena bombing: lessons learnt from a mass casualty incident. BMJ Mil Health. 2020;166:72–5.
50. Brewin CR, Fuchkan N, Huntley Z, et al. Outreach and screening following the 2005 London bombings: usage and outcomes. Psychol Med. 2010;40:2049–57.
51. Haga JM, Stene LE, Wentzel-Larsen T, et al. Early postdisaster health outreach to modern families: a cross-sectional study. BMJ Open. 2015;5:e009402.
52. Dyb G, Jensen T, Glad KA, et al. Early outreach to survivors of the shootings in Norway on the 22nd of July 2011. Eur J Psychotraumatol. 5 https://doi.org/10.3402/ejpt.v5.23523.
53. Brewin CR, Scragg P, Robertson M, et al. Promoting mental health following the London bombings: a screen and treat approach. J Trauma Stress. 2008;21:3–8.
54. Wiström ED, Stene LE, Dyb G. Following the Utøya attack—who received early assistance? Tidsskrift for Den norske legeforening. 2016; https://doi.org/10.4045/tidsskr.15.0691.
55. Stevens GJ, Dunsmore JC, Agho KE, et al. Coping support factors among Australians affected by terrorism: 2002 Bali bombing survivors speak. Med J Aust. 2013;199:772–5.
56. Hobfoll SE, Watson P, Bell CC, et al. Five essential elements of immediate and mid–term mass trauma intervention: empirical evidence. Psychiatry Interpers Biolog Processes. 2007;70:283–315.
57. Haga JM, Thoresen S, Stene LE, et al. Healthcare to parents of young terrorism survivors: a registry-based study in Norway. BMJ Open. 2017;7:e018358.
58. Bengel J, Becker-Nehring K, Hillebrecht J. Early psychological interventions. In: Trauma Sequelae. Berlin, Heidelberg: Springer; 2022. p. 175–202.
59. Garfield R. Commentary: the evolving role of nurses in terrorism and war. Am J Infect Control. 2003;31:163–7.
60. Dieltjens T, Moonens I, Van Praet K, et al. A systematic literature search on psychological first aid: lack of evidence to develop guidelines. PLoS One. 2014;9:e114714.
61. Kouvatsou Z, Degermedgoglou G, Karamagioli E, et al. Psychological first aid training of police officers. J Police Crim Psychol. 2022;37:856–62.
62. Pandya A. A review and retrospective analysis of mental health services provided after the September 11 attacks. Can J Psychiatry. 2013;58:128–34.
63. Shultz JM, Forbes D. Psychological first aid. Disaster Health. 2014;2:3–12.

64. Wang L, Norman I, Edleston V, et al. The effectiveness and implementation of psychological first aid as a therapeutic intervention after trauma: an integrative review. Trauma Violence Abuse. 2024;25:2638–56.
65. Tan JT, Gan RK, Alsua C, et al. Psychological first aid by AI: proof-of-concept and comparative performance of ChatGPT-4 and Gemini in different disaster scenarios. J Clin Psychol. 2025;81:726–38.
66. Koda M, Horinouchi T, Oya N, et al. Effectiveness of psychological first aid in infectious disease pandemics: an overview of systematic reviews. Psychiatry Clin Neurosci Rep. 2023;2 https://doi.org/10.1002/pcn5.107.
67. Figueroa RA, Cortés PF, Miller C, et al. The effect of a single session of psychological first aid in the emergency department on PTSD and depressive symptoms three months post-intervention: results of a randomised controlled trial. Eur J Psychotraumatol. 2024;15 https://doi.org/10.1080/20008066.2024.2364443.
68. Ghuman SJ, Brackbill RM, Stellman SD, et al. Unmet mental health care need 10–11 years after the 9/11 terrorist attacks: 2011–2012 results from the World Trade Center Health Registry. BMC Public Health. 2014;14:491.
69. Van Overmeire R. The myth of psychological debriefings during the corona pandemic. J Glob Health. 2020;10 https://doi.org/10.7189/jogh.10.020344.
70. Knobler HY, Nachshoni T, Jaffe E, et al. Psychological guidelines for a medical team debriefing after a stressful event. Mil Med. 2007;172:581–5.
71. Eppich WJ, Mullan PC, Brett-Fleegler M, et al. "Let's Talk About It": translating lessons from health care simulation to clinical event debriefings and coaching conversations. Clin Pediatr Emerg Med. 2016;17:200–11.
72. Kagee A. Concerns about the effectiveness of critical incident stress debriefing in ameliorating stress reactions. Crit Care. 2002;6:88.
73. Tran DV, North CS. The association between dissatisfaction with debriefing and post-traumatic stress disorder (PTSD) in rescue and recovery workers for the Oklahoma City Bombing. Disaster Med Public Health Prep. 2018;12:718–22.
74. Mansdorf IJ. Psychological interventions following terrorist attacks. Br Med Bull. 2008;88:7–22.
75. Dückers MLA, Witteveen AB, Bisson JI, et al. The association between disaster vulnerability and post-disaster psychosocial service delivery across Europe. Adm Policy Ment Health Ment Health Serv Res. 2017;44:470–9.
76. Pfefferbaum B. Disasters in the 21st century: lessons from project liberty. Psychiatr Serv. 2006;57:1251.
77. Tharp PAT, Constans PJI, Yin LR, et al. Service provision in disaster preparation, response, and recovery for individuals with predisaster mental illness. Am J Disaster Med. 2012;7:171–4.
78. van der Velden PG, Contino C, Das M, et al. To what extent do post-traumatic mental health and other problems reflect pre-existing problems? Findings from the prospective comparative population-based VICTIMS-study. Int J Soc Psychiatry. 2023;69:841–52.
79. French P, Barrett A, Allsopp K, et al. Psychological screening of adults and young people following the Manchester Arena incident. BJPsych Open. 2019;5:e85.
80. Steenkamp MM, Dickstein BD, Salters-Pedneault K, et al. Trajectories of PTSD symptoms following sexual assault: Is resilience the modal outcome? J Trauma Stress. 2012;25:469–74.
81. Elklit A, Christiansen DM. ASD and PTSD in rape victims. J Interpers Violence. 2010;25:1470–88.
82. Covell NH, Essock SM, Felton CJ, et al. Characteristics of project liberty clients that predicted referrals to intensive mental health services. Psychiatr Serv. 2006;57:1313–5.
83. Covell NH, Donahue SA, Allen G, et al. Use of project liberty counseling services over time by individuals in various risk categories. Psychiatr Serv. 2006;57:1268–70.
84. Donahue SA, Lanzara CB, Felton CJ, et al. Project liberty: New York's crisis counseling program created in the aftermath of September 11, 2001. Psychiatr Serv. 2006;57:1253–8.

85. Neria Y, Markowitz JC, Amsalem D, et al. Israeli mental health in the aftermath of the October 7 terrorist attack: risks, challenges, and recommendations. Isr J Health Policy Res. 2025;14:25.
86. Kerslake B. *The Kerslake report: an independent review into the preparedness for, and emergency response to, the Manchester Arena attack on 22nd May 2017.* Manchester, https://www.jesip.org.uk/uploads/media/Documents%20Products/Kerslake_Report_Manchester_Are.pdf (2018, accessed 21 February 2026).
87. van Herpen MM, Dückers MLA, Schaap R, et al. Online one-stop shop for disaster response services after the MH17 airplane crash: an evaluation study. Front Public Health. 2022;10 https://doi.org/10.3389/fpubh.2022.832840.
88. Lynch O, Argomaniz J. Victims of terrorism and political violence: identity, needs, and service delivery in Northern Ireland and Great Britain. Terrorism Political Violence. 2017;29:464–82.
89. Bosmans MWG, Plevier C, Schutz F, et al. The impact of a terrorist attack: survivors' health, functioning and need for support following the 2019 Utrecht tram shooting 6 and 18 months post-attack. Front Psychol. 2022;13 https://doi.org/10.3389/fpsyg.2022.981280.
90. Drury J, Stancombe J, Williams R, et al. Survivors' experiences of informal social support in coping and recovering after the 2017 Manchester Arena bombing. BJPsych Open. 2022;8:e124.
91. Gomes C, McGuire TG, Foster MJ, et al. Did project liberty displace community-based medicaid services in New York? Psychiatr Serv. 2006;57:1309–12.
92. Skøt L, Jeppesen T, Mellentin AI, et al. Accessibility of medical and psychosocial services following disasters and other traumatic events: experiences of Deaf and hard-of-hearing individuals in Denmark. Disabil Rehabil. 2017;39:2468–76.
93. Cyhlarova E, Knapp M, Mays N. Responding to the mental health consequences of the 2015–2016 terrorist attacks in Tunisia, Paris and Brussels: implementation and treatment experiences in the United Kingdom. J Health Serv Res Policy. 2020;25:172–80.
94. Gobin M, Rubin GJ, Albert I, et al. Outcomes of Mental Health Screening for United Kingdom Nationals Affected by the 2015–2016 Terrorist Attacks in Tunisia, Paris, and Brussels. J Trauma Stress. 2018;31:471–9.
95. Call JA, Pfefferbaum B. Lessons from the first two years of Project Heartland, Oklahoma's mental health response to the 1995 bombing. Psychiatr Serv. 1999;50:953–5.
96. Jackson CT, Allen G, Essock SM, et al. Clusters of event reactions among recipients of project liberty mental health counseling. Psychiatr Serv. 2006;57:1271–6.
97. Frank RG, Pindyck T, Donahue SA, et al. Impact of a media campaign for disaster mental health counseling in post-September 11 New York. Psychiatr Serv. 2006;57:1304–8.
98. Stene LE, Glad KA, Stensland SØ, et al. Proactive psychosocial follow-up of youth exposed to a terrorist attack: longitudinal study linking interviews and register-based data. BJPsych Open. 2025;11:e48.
99. Wagner AW. Cognitive-behavioral therapy for posttraumatic stress disorder: applications to injured trauma survivors. Semin Clin Neuropsychiatry 2003; 8.: as1084361203000182.
100. Walser RD, Ruzek JI, Naugle AE, et al. Disaster and terrorism: cognitive-behavioral interventions. Prehosp Disaster Med. 2004;19:54–63.
101. Donahue SA, Jackson CT, Shear KM, et al. Outcomes of enhanced counseling services provided to adults through project liberty. Psychiatr Serv. 2006;57:1298–303.
102. Bryant RA, Ekasawin S, Chakrabhand S, et al. A randomized controlled effectiveness trial of cognitive behavior therapy for post-traumatic stress disorder in terrorist-affected people in Thailand. World Psychiatry. 2011;10:205–9.
103. Gillespie K, Duffy M, Hackmann A, et al. Community based cognitive therapy in the treatment of post-traumatic stress disorder following the Omagh bomb. Behav Res Ther. 2002;40:345–57.
104. Chemtob CM, Nakashima JP, Hamada RS. Psychosocial Intervention for postdisaster trauma symptoms in elementary school children. Arch Pediatr Adolesc Med. 2002;156:211.

105. Kazdin A. A school based psychosocial intervention was effective in children with persistent post-disaster trauma symptoms. Evidence Based Mental Health. 2002;5:76.
106. Tol WA, Komproe IH, Susanty D, et al. School-based mental health intervention for children affected by political violence in Indonesia. JAMA. 2008;300:655.
107. Miller L. Psychotherapeutic interventions for survivors of terrorism. Am J Psychother. 2004;58:1–16.
108. Jackson CT, Allen G, Essock SM, et al. Clients' satisfaction with project liberty counseling services. Psychiatr Serv. 2006;57:1316–9.
109. Possick C, Shamai M, Sadeh RA. Healing the social self: how parents whose children were killed in terror attacks construct the experience of help. Community Ment Health J. 2014;50:487–96.
110. Kärki FU. Norway's 2011 terror attacks: alleviating national trauma with a large-scale proactive intervention model. Psychiatr Serv. 2015;66:910–2.
111. Van Overmeire R, Vesentini L, Van Keer R-L, et al. Working experiences of airport employees after a terrorist attack in Belgium: a qualitative study. Int J Dis Risk Reduct. 2021;64:102515.
112. Stene LE, Dyb G. Research participation after terrorism: an open cohort study of survivors and parents after the 2011 Utøya attack in Norway. BMC Res Notes. 2016;9:57.
113. Sulaiman-Hill R, Porter R, Schluter P, et al. Research following trauma in minority ethnic and faith communities: lessons from a study of the psychosocial sequelae of the Christchurch mosque terror attacks. BJPsych Open. 2024;10:e27.
114. North CS. The Oklahoma City bombing study and methodological issues in longitudinal disaster mental health research. J Trauma Dissociation. 2005;6:27–35.
115. North CS. A tale of two studies of two disasters: Comparing psychosocial responses to disaster among Oklahoma City bombing survivors and Hurricane Katrina evacuees. Rehabil Psychol. 2010;55:241–6.
116. Gouweloos J, Dückers M, te Brake H, et al. Psychosocial care to affected citizens and communities in case of CBRN incidents: a systematic review. Environ Int. 2014;72:46–65.
117. Reifels L, Pietrantoni L, Prati G, et al. Lessons learned about psychosocial responses to disaster and mass trauma: an international perspective. Eur J Psychotraumatol. 2013;4 https://doi.org/10.3402/ejpt.v4i0.22897.
118. Murthy R. Mental health of survivors of 1984 Bhopal disaster: a continuing challenge. Ind Psychiatry J. 2014;23:86.
119. Schäfer I, Hopchet M, Vandamme N, et al. Trauma and trauma care in Europe. Eur J Psychotraumatol. 2018;9 https://doi.org/10.1080/20008198.2018.1556553.
120. Tolstoy L, Kahn A, Maude L, et al. Resurrection. Alfred A. Knopf; 2025.
121. Nilsen LG, Thoresen S, Wentzel-Larsen T, et al. Trust after terror: institutional trust among young terror survivors and their parents after the 22nd of July terrorist attack on Utøya Island, Norway. Front Psychol. 2019;10 https://doi.org/10.3389/fpsyg.2019.02819.
122. Home Office Victims of Terrorism Unit. *Review of support for victims and survivors of terrorism*, https://www.gov.uk/government/publications/review-of-support-for-victims-and-survivors-of-terrorism/review-of-support-for-victims-and-survivors-of-terrorism. 2025. Accessed 22 Feb 2026.

# Chapter 10
# Remembering Memories: Trauma and Recognition

## 10.1 Trauma: A History of Amnesia and Rediscovery [1]

The Ise Jingu Shinto shrine in Japan is rebuilt every 20 years, roughly the time of a generation [2]. The knowledge of trauma has a similar pattern: every generation seems to have to find recognition for the idea that trauma can cause mental health issues. Knowledge about trauma often has been deliberately forgotten throughout time, and every time it had to be rediscovered [1, 3].

When people started suing railway companies when they were experiencing mental health issues after train disasters, some doctors suggested they were all malingers trying to get money by pretending to have suffered due to the crash [4].

After the First World War, some soldiers returned home and found that they could not find a job, had no social relationships left, and no prospects, yet a part of the population felt that the shellshock the soldiers suffered from was due to their own personal failure [5].

During the Second World War, millions of soldiers suffered from mental health issues due to exposure to war. A psychiatrist named Edward Strecker wrote that these men are simply immature, and that there is a need for grown-up men, because else democracy would fall apart [6]. Indeed, throughout the end of the nineteenth century, and through the twentieth century, mental health was a threat against ideas of patriotism and nationalism [5].

As Haruki Murakami, the Japanese author, writes in "Killing Commendatore" in his many attempts to bring the Japanese war experience more to the forefront: "*In fact, though, it was clear to everyone why Uncle Tsuguhiko had taken his own life—his war experience ruined his nerves and wrecked him psychologically. I mean here*

---

Parts of this chapter are based on my doctoral thesis, defended in 2021. Van Overmeire, R. (2021). The association between exposure to terrorist attacks and mental health in Belgium. [PhD Thesis, Vrije Universiteit Brussel]. VUB Press. https://cris.vub.be/ws/portalfiles/portal/86873200/1_PDFsam_Van_Overmeire_Roel_PhD_thesis_20.12.2021.pdf.



R. Van Overmeire, *Terrorism, Mental Health and Aftercare*,
https://doi.org/10.1007/978-3-032-31560-1_10

*was a delicate young man of twenty, whose entire world was playing the piano, thrown into the bloodbath of the Nanjing campaign, surrounded by heaps of corpses. [...] In that deeply militaristic society, people like my uncle were dismissed as lacking courage, or patriotism, or strength of character. In wartime Japan, such 'weakness' was neither understood nor accepted. So the family buried what had happened, as evidence of their shame*" [7]. That shame is not exclusive for military societies; it is present in any democracy as well.

**A Report from the Second World War**
General Eisenhower commissioned a report after the Second World war on why soldiers were unable to fight due to mental health problems. The commission reported "*There is no such thing as 'getting used to combat'... Most men were ineffective after 180 or even 140 days... The general consensus was that a man reached his peak of effectiveness in the first 90 days of combat, that after that his efficiency began to fall out*" [8].

The process to get recognition for trauma is often long and difficult, but as Judith Herman wrote "*The conflict between the will to deny horrible events and the will to proclaim them aloud is the central dialectic of psychological trauma. People who have survived atrocities often tell their stories in a highly emotional, contradictory, and fragmented manner which undermines their credibility and thereby serves the twin imperatives of truth-telling and secrecy. When the truth is finally recognized, survivors can begin their recovery.*" [1] The recognition of the trauma is essential for survivors in their recovery. Or in other words: recognition makes a horrible event into a trauma that society agrees is a trauma.

In this chapter, the importance, and difficulties, of recognition of terrorism survivors will be discussed, and attention will be drawn to the importance of it for public health policy.

This need for recognition has two reasons.

## 10.2 Legal Need for Recognition

First, a legal, financial, or even administrative reason. Recognition of being a victim can lead to the feeling of justice, truth, but also economic compensation and political representation [9]. A survivor of terrorism constantly needs to prove their damages, whether physical or mental—though often, proving physical injuries is much easier than mental health injuries, which is a common frustration of survivors [10, 11].

Due to the fragmentation of services, they need to retell and relive their story every time [12]. A recognition already helps a lot in terms of relieving the burden on survivors. Additionally, a recognition also can lead to a form of compensation. This can for example finance the therapy victims might need or simply be a compensation for having to be exposed to terrorist attacks that were aimed at the state and not them personally.

Secondly, for social reasons, which will be discussed more below.

## 10.3 Social Need for Recognition

### *10.3.1 Redefining the Social Role*

Whether it is victims who suffer from post-traumatic stress disorder (PTSD), or loved ones who lost someone in the attacks, terrorism can affect the social role someone has [13]. For example, in one case, a mother did not want to recognize the effect the attacks had on her mental health, because she did not want to lose her role as mother [11, 14]. The importance of recognition of being a victim therefore helps with the identity building as a victim [12], which is important in how a survivor of terrorism sees themselves moving forward from the trauma [15].

This recognition of being a victim also helps to create "victimhood,"[1] namely the creation of identity based on the harm done to a group [9]. This collective identity derived from a collective trauma provides victims with a purpose, values, and a collective worth [16]. It is through this collective identity, this victimhood, that victim support groups can be made, which are of the upmost importance for long-term social support [11, 17, 18].

Thus, this creation of victimhood is very important in terms of public health, as it can lead to social support groups. In addition, it can lead to social acknowledgment.

### *10.3.2 Social Acknowledgement*

This social acknowledgement is, in short, the societal view of the trauma experience of someone. In this case, it is the view of the community and society in general of the victim and their trauma [19–21]. For example, sexual assault can be viewed as taboo, and victim blaming is often not uncommon. In fact, studies also show that sexual assault is the least disclosed trauma in some countries [22]. Similarly, the mental health issues one might have after terrorist attacks can be viewed with a certain disbelief and lack of understanding [11]. In fact, victims have to often face

[1] In other chapters, victimhood was also mentioned, and often in the context of it being typical for Western societies. In this chapter, the meaning of "victimhood" refers to a social, group process, while other chapters referred to a "cultural" victimhood.

people who do not understand that they have not "moved on" [12]. As such, mental health issues due to trauma are breaking a "norm," and a way of acceptance of this breaking of norm is due to understanding that this is due to the exposure to attacks [11, 23].

Not surprisingly therefore, when there is social acknowledgement in a society, this acts as a buffer against the development of PTSD, as there is more understanding and sympathy for what the person is going through [19].

Recognition can lead to this social acknowledgement, as it shows that the political level acknowledges that victims of terrorism can experiences problems that (1) are real and scientifically acknowledged and (2) that these mental health issues are not their own responsibility, but were done to them by others [24].

### *10.3.3 Societal Belief*

Another important consequence of the political act of recognition is that it also allows victims to make meaning of an event and begin reparations, not just financial, but also emotionally [25]. As noted by Erikson [26] and other authors, trauma can cause one's belief of humanity, of the lawfulness of society, of one's trust, to crumble, making sure that all future social relationships are based on this principle of distrust, belief of unlawfulness, etc. Solomon [27] called it *"the shattering of believes someone has about the world."*

Thus, recognition allows victims to again believe in the lawfulness of the society they live in [28]. Not doing so is effectively creating social exclusion, because society, as represented by the democratic chosen government, states that one's experience is not terrible enough that society should begin reparations [28]. Which might add to the idea that the mental health issues of those directly exposed are due ill-will, weak character, etc., which, as the introduction of this chapter showed, are accusations that have been repeated time and again.

### *10.3.4 Consequences of Non-recognition*

When an event is not recognized in all its forms, the mental health burden is not the fault of the attacks, but the survivors own lack of will to come through. A survivor has to deal not only with the tragedy of trauma, but also with the tragedy of people not believing the tragedy of the trauma [29, 30]. As Solomon [27] put it: throughout history, people with trauma are blamed for having experienced the trauma [29, 30].

Without recognition of being a survivor of the attack, it is more difficult to get understanding and empathy from others. After all, the evidence that one is a survivor of the attack mainly comes down to memories of the individual and the disclosure of the trauma. Public health policy will always be limited if it does not recognize survivors.

Yet, there are two major issues for policy with regard to recognition. First: what is a survivor of terrorism? Second: unwillingness of policy to recognize the survivor.

**Recognition for All?**
Any form of recognition of victims and victimhood is a choice, and any such choice will exclude some [9]. This is important to victims of disasters, as their victimhood might be affected if people are included in the recognition they feel do not deserve to be there. As such, some victims will be suspicious of others receiving reimbursements or compensations. As one survivor stated:

*"A colleague that hears that you can get compensationif you have problems, and suddenly she gets problems and demands a compensationfor damages ... Now, I'm no doctor, I didn't study for that, and I won't, but I think that's weird."* [31]

In fact, this need for "purity" in being a victim seems to be connected with PTSD. PTSD and trauma are so closely linked to each in the public's eye that sometimes the search for recognition begins with the recognition of having PTSD. Having PTSD is seen as being evidence of being a victim of trauma, or in this case, of the attack [32–34].

This way PTSD is used as a way to show that someone is a victim is probably more a Western phenomenon where PTSD and trauma are often used colloquial, and where therapy-speak is more common. As such, stating one has PTSD becomes equivalent to being a victim or survivor of trauma [34].

The importance of naming an experience in terms of mental health issues is not new and common in the history of trauma. For example, soldiers during the First World War were able to discuss their fears because of the naming of their experiences under the umbrella term "shellshock," despite the diagnoses used in the war itself were neurasthenia and hysteria [5]. This was also because "shellshock" indicated an organic origin, to avoid the stigma of mental health issues, which were often associated with weakness or insanity [ 5].

## 10.4 What Is a Victim? What Is a Survivor?

Throughout this book, the term "survivor" was used. Generally, survivors of terrorism prefer that term: survivor, instead of victim, as victims are, in their view, people who were killed [35]. International literature still uses mainly "victim," as do many psychosocial disaster plans [35, 36]. In this chapter, the terms "victim" and "survivor" will be employed interchangeably.

Whether survivor or victim, what is someone like that in relation to terrorism? As mentioned in Chap. 1, to define terrorism is a difficult task. What a victim or survivor of terrorism is therefore even more difficult [35, 37]. It remains unclear legally what a survivor of terrorism is, and what it actually means [37].

A side-effect of the state making sure who is a victim and who is not is that it is an unequal affair, in the sense that not all victims of terrorism will receive the same [9]. For example, if terrorism-victim is defined as such that someone needs to either have been present at the attacks, or have lost someone in the attacks, those that are partner to someone simply wounded in the attack are not seen as victim of the attacks, despite the possible loss to income, social life, and mental health issues related to this. As such, defining is choosing.

There are clear examples after terrorism where this categorization of victimhood causes problems, or barriers [38].

**An Attempt at Defining "Victims of Terrorism"**

A United Nations Special Rapporteur on the promotion and protection of human rights and fundamental freedoms while countering terrorism provided a definition of victims of terrorism, splitting the term up into four categories [37].

1. Direct victims of terrorism, such as people who suffered physical or psychological injuries due to terrorism.
2. Secondary victims of terrorism, such as immediate family, or people dependent on direct victims. This would be, for example, the families of the victims of the Mumbai attacks shortly discussed in Chap. 2, who had to change their entire lives because they were dependent on the victims for financial security [39, 40]. Under the DSM-5 definition, these would be also considered as those exposed to trauma [41].
3. Indirect victims of terrorism, which is the public at large, or people who viewed it on television or social media, though this also includes eyewitnesses.
4. "Potential victims of terrorism," which refers to the legal obligation of the State under article six of the International Covenant on Civil and Political Rights.

A problem of this definition seems to be that everyone can be a victim in some degree of terrorism, and that it differentiates between direct and secondary victims, even though it seems that people who dependent on someone for their livelihood, or suffer from mental health issues due to a terrorist attack against a loved one, could be seen as primary victims.

The United Nations Model Provisions states that a "victim of terrorism" can have either individually or collectively suffered harm, whether physical or mental, economic loss, substantial impairment of fundamental rights.

## 10.5 Barriers to Recognition

Governments generally are not very eager to recognize events as traumatic events or disasters, as this is, among other reasons, admission of guilt, and might open the door to legal repercussion, and possibly more victim compensations [25, 30, 42].

Additionally, the idea of victim compensations has social consequences. While survivors of a storm are not always seen as "heroic," survivors of terrorist attacks are sometimes seen heroes, or as people who saw "the face of evil" and came through [25]. It is even the way in which books by survivors are marketed: there are lessons to learn from their traumatic experience [30]. This image of heroism changes quickly the moment compensations come into play, despite compensations being at the centre of recognition, as there is no recognition without compensation [25]. From the moment compensations are mentioned, everything can become questioned about the victim, even the essence of their victimhood: the experience of the attack. Questions are raised such as "Were they really there at the attacks? Do they deserve such compensations? Why them, and not us?" [30]

For example, a survivor of terrorism who sought out help stated:

> *"The hours I was with the psychologists (of the police) I still got paid. And the commissioner called me like 'Hey, it better be over with profiting, you don't have any right to do that!'"* [31]

## 10.6 The Campaign for Recognition

A so-called lay history of a terrorist attack begins immediately after the attacks, in the sharing of emotions and events [43, 44]. Collective memories of attacks therefore start from the moment victims share their experiences of the attack [45].

However, this does not automatically translate to recognition.

**Narratives of Terrorist Attacks and PTSD**

Victims with PTSD often provide different narratives of the attacks than those without PTSD. One notable difference is that those without PTSD will often tell their experiences of the attacks in plural ("we"), while those with PTSD more often singular ("I") [45, 46]. Some studies also show that memories of those with PTSD will more often include references to violence and death (e.g. "blood", "bullet", "wound"...). Finally, victims with PTSD more often have less "control" over their narrative, with it changing, or some details being more highlighted [45]. Indeed, the paradox of remembering trauma is that is can be focussed on very specific aspects of the trauma, that can be described to a high degree, but at the same time, the victim might not remember a lot of other aspects [1].

The "campaign for recognition," and the time waiting for problems to be taken seriously, has been called "slow violence." That, in short, means that the disaster has passed, but the disaster still acts violently on the victims, while the bureaucracy works slowly (or the government does not want to act too much upon the issues due to the previously mentioned reasons) [30, 42]. As such, survivors, sometimes bonded by the collective trauma, start campaigning for recognition.

**The Campaign for Recognition in Belgium**

The lack of recognition for survivors of the 2016 Belgium attack resulted in two victim support groups, VEurope and Life4Brussels [47, 48]. In the years following, there has been an increase in laws to help victims of the terrorist attacks in Belgium. Five years after the attacks, there has been more attention for the attacks, with programs on the television channel VRT on the attacks and the mental health impact on the victims (e.g. "And then it was silent" (Original in Dutch: "En toen was het stil")) [49], and ten years later, one contact point was made for victims of terrorism [50].

Jeffrey Alexander wrote about how a trauma "becomes" a trauma in a cultural sense [51]. In other words, why is one tragedy viewed as a tragedy while another is not? In short, through a campaign that raised awareness, a large impulse in society to be "outraged" by an event or a type of event [30].

Such campaigns have occurred for even interpersonal trauma. For example, the 1970s and 1980s brought forth a campaign for the recognition of sexual assault and child abuse. Importantly, sexual assault now also fell under the newly described post-traumatic stress disorder (PTSD) diagnosis, made in 1980 in DSM-III [1]. This certainly was not because of a lack of knowledge of sexual abuse nor child abuse. In fact, even in the late nineteenth century, early twentieth century, surveys showed that child abuse might be a lot higher than was expected [1, 52].

Another example [51] is the recognition of the trauma of the Holocaust. In the years after World War Two, the Holocaust was largely ignored in favour of the military victories and the tendency from both society and victims to "try and forget" [1], yet something of this scale is not easily forgotten. Whether through the works of Primo Levi, the trial of Eichmann in 1961, or TV-shows such as "Holocaust" [30], more awareness of the fate of Jewish people in the Holocaust was created in society, yet while the Jewish fate in the Holocaust was highlighted, the campaign for recognizing the fate of homosexuals of Roma's was not. As such, sometimes campaigns succeed, sometimes they fail.

**Socioeconomic Aspects of Recognition Campaigns**

Campaigns for recognition after disasters can be limited by socioeconomic factors. Schutt [53] gives as example the flooding of a river in a town. While the mayor of the town explains the disaster is outside his control (as the mayor, to our knowledge, has no control of the elements nor nature), the damages

(continued)

(continued)

such a disasters havocs are socially controlled, and will often affect the socio-economic weaker groups. While obviously these groups often have less financial capital to rebuild their lives, the point by Schutt [53] is actually that, epidemiologically speaking, disasters tend to hit people in weak social positions. Why? While the mayor of the town that was flooded stated that he could not control nature, the issue was not his lack of supernatural abilities; it was that all the poor people lived right next to the river, because land is cheaper there, precisely because the river tended to flood. Similarly, Hurricane Katrina flooded poor black neighbourhoods more than those of the white middle-class population [30, 54]. As Bullard writes: "*what many people often call 'natural' disasters are in fact acts of social injustice perpetuated by government and business on the poor, people of color, the disabled, the elderly, the homeless, those who are transit dependent, and non-drivers— groups least able to withstand such disasters*" [55].

While some argue that the meaning of disasters has changed, going from "Acts of God" to events with human responsibility to them, with emphasis on vulnerability [56], it might as well be that the reason disaster have changed in meaning due to those being affected by trauma were more often those without a voice to do so, and that only later in the twentieth century this changed. After all, even studies from the first decade of the twentieth century showed that victims of disasters suffered from mental health issues after disasters [57]. Indeed, public recognition of the possible impact of disasters came much later in the century, but a lack of recognition does not mean that there was no mental health impact. Similarly, in the late nineteenth century sexual abuse of children was well-documented in France, yet general recognition to protect children from such abuse came much later as well [1, 57].

Thus, before being recognized as a survivor of terrorism, the importance of the event of the terrorist attack needs to be recognized. If a policy, or culture, dismisses the importance of the terrorist attack, being a survivor of it has no cultural nor legal meaning.

## 10.7 How Then to Achieve It?

Sociologist C. Mills [ 58], while not writing about trauma, provided a general point of the importance of collective action. Any issue, whether trauma or not, will never lead to collective action unless the personal issue (in this case, the exposure to terrorist attacks) can be extrapolated to being an issue that many people face. For example, if someone is sexually assaulted by their superior, this is a "personal" problem, but to make this into a collective and societal issue, it needs to be recognized as a "personal" problem many people face. Similarly, the issues soldiers faced during the Vietnam war were reframed as being an issue of the American people [30]. In fact, while the diagnosis of PTSD came mainly from the experience of Vietnam veterans, to give it more strength, it was made broader, more general, and not "specific" for veterans of war [59]. Hence this is why the trauma definition was made broad, and could be applied to any number of non-war related traumas.

As such, it is important that victims align themselves to a "master narrative" [9]. For terrorism survivors, this can be aspects such as the value of democracy and freedom, or the overall wave of religious extremist attacks. Victims, once banded together, need to a waken a political consciousness, use the master narrative to explain what they have gone through (e.g. coming to the point that simply saying "9/11" has meaning in itself on what they have gone through), and showcase how their suffering is part of the overall story. For example, the war on terror needs to be linked with the mental health issues one has, and terrorism needs to be seen as not just consisting of "terrorist," but also of victims. After this, political mobilization and recognition follow [9, 24].

Sometimes recognition occurs fast, sometimes it is a long process of "slow violence."

**Failing Campaigns**
There are many terrorism recognition campaigns that fail or might not even start. If terrorism is a regular occurrence, its exceptionality is not clear, and thus the recognition of it as well. Furthermore, the creation of "victimhood" is often more present in democratic countries, that allow that freedom of expression, while in countries that do not allow this, this is difficult to create [9]. However, sometimes recognition of a mass trauma might also be limited by other factors, such as socioeconomic factors, or race. For example, after Hurricane Katrina, the majority of black victims were portrayed as anti-social in the media, which might have influenced the disaster relief of the government [60].

## 10.8 Memorials and Memory

Remembering terrorist attacks is a social act [16, 45]. Memorials and official recognition showcase that the state wants the terrorist attacks to be part of the national history and of the collective memory of the state. Remembering therefore becomes an official way of showing "deviance," to use Emile Durkheim's term [61]: it is showcasing what is out of the ordinary, and by showcasing this, reinforces what is seen as the normality of life. As such, the memory of a terrorist attack becomes a "usable past": it showcases what the society is, and what should be done when threats occur, and how to respond effectively [16, 44]. As such, it provides future victims of terrorism a narrative, a way of gaining quicker recognition for themselves, from the state, but also from their social support [9, 24].

Trauma loses its edge of pain as time goes on, and when recognized, changes from a history of senseless loss to lessons [16]. A memorial is therefore an official representation of the lessons learned, and can such also become a way of creating hope out of misery [62]. Naturally, due to the importance of this, it is no wonder therefore that sometimes the form and place of memorials can be a point of twist [31, 63].

## 10.9 Public Health Implications

A report on victims of terrorism and reparations ends with "[...] *there is no justice without reparation*" [64]. In a broader sense, indeed, victims of terrorism might feel there is no justice in the world at all. Survivors will blame the government for not protecting them, and their individual grief following the terrorist attacks flows into a broader narrative about the nation [ 38]. A lack of attention for their plight or their collective trauma can influence the meaning-making processes, yet disasters can also be the beginning of new communities, hope and strength, and post-traumatic growth [26, 65–67].

It is here that public health policy is deeply linked with recognition. The previous chapters noted the importance of community approaches and social support. This chapter shows that a lack of recognition can hamper the community approach and social support in the long run, since there is no example for communities or social support to believe that the mental health issues a victim might go through are in any way linked to the attack, and it is exactly this social support, as well as communities, which are the most important in the recovery process of victims [68–70]. Additionally, recognition of being a victim of terrorism provides the basis for the new social identity discussed earlier, and this alone also provides the basis for resilience and post-traumatic growth [71].

As mentioned, this has been the struggle of those that suffered from trauma throughout time: whether it is doctors stating that those who experienced man-made disasters were mostly malingers [4, 72], soldiers being called unpatriotic because of their mental health issues after combat [5], or simply terrorism survivors being called profiteers [14, 31].

While there can certainly be critique on the therapy-speak [34], victimhood-culture [73], and other aspects related to recognition, from a public health perspective, which is the driving force of this book, recognition is important for the recovery process on a community and social level.

## 10.10 Conclusion

This chapter is the last of this book as it completes the cycle of the survivor. The survivor of a terrorist attack experiences the attacks, might develop mental health issues, and then needs to face recovery, in the form of social interactions and healthcare, and finally needs to have societal "approval" of their experience.

This chapter aimed at providing a view into the importance of recognition, while avoiding diving too deep into the sociological complexities of victimhood and recognition. The aim was of this chapter, while being politically and socially driven research, to show the connection of this importance to public health, as it fulfills both parts of the term.

## References

1. Herman J. Trauma and recovery. New York: Basic Books; 1992.
2. Wang D. Breakneck: China's quest to engineer the future. London: Allen Lane; 2025.
3. Young A. The Harmony of illusions: inventing post-traumatic stress disorder. Princeton, NJ: Princeton University Press; 1995.
4. Caplan E. Trains and trauma in the American gilded age. In: Micale MS, Lerner P, editors. Traumatic pasts. Cambridge: Cambridge University Press; 2001.
5. Leese P. Shell shock: traumatic neurosis and the British soldiers of the First World War. Palgrave; 2002.
6. Strecker EA. Their mothers' sons; the psychiatrist examines an American problem. Lippincott; 1946.
7. Murakami H, Gabriel P, Goossen T. Killing commendatore. Harvill Secker; 2019.
8. Bartemeier LH, Kubie LS, Menninger KA, et al. Combat exhaustion. J Nerv Ment Dis. 1946;104:358–89.
9. Jacoby TA. A theory of victimhood: politics, conflict and the construction of victim-based identity. Millennium J Int Stud. 2015;43:511–30.
10. Bos JN, Farmer J, Nelson S. The good, the bad, and the ugly: victims of terrorism experiences with government responses and policy. Int Rev Vict. 2026; https://doi.org/10.1177/02697580261416534.
11. Van Overmeire R, Van Keer R, Bilsen J. Impact of terrorist attacks on social relationships. Clin Psychol Psychother. 2021;28:1472–81.
12. Lynch O, Argomaniz J. Victims of terrorism and political violence: identity, needs, and service delivery in Northern Ireland and Great Britain. Terrorism Political Violence. 2017;29:464–82.
13. Stevenson M, Achille M, Liben S, et al. Understanding how bereaved parents cope with their grief to inform the services provided to them. Qual Health Res. 2017;27:649–64.
14. Van Overmeire R, Muysewinkel E, Van Keer R-L, et al. Victims of the terrorist attacks in Belgium and professional mental health aid barriers: a qualitative study. Front Psychiatry. 2021;12 https://doi.org/10.3389/fpsyt.2021.638272.
15. Meredith VM. Victim identity and respect for human dignity: a terminological analysis. Int Rev Red Cross. 2009;91:259–77.
16. Hirschberger G. Collective trauma and the social construction of meaning. Front Psychol. 2018;9 https://doi.org/10.3389/fpsyg.2018.01441.
17. Aoun SM, Breen LJ, Rumbold B, et al. Matching response to need: what makes social networks fit for providing bereavement support? PLoS One. 2019;14:e0213367.

18. Aoun SM, Breen LJ, White I, et al. What sources of bereavement support are perceived helpful by bereaved people and why? Empirical evidence for the compassionate communities approach. Palliat Med. 2018;32:1378–88.
19. Maercker A, Müller J. Social acknowledgment as a victim or survivor: a scale to measure a recovery factor of PTSD. J Trauma Stress. 2004;17:345–51.
20. Maercker A, Hecker T. Broadening perspectives on trauma and recovery: a socio-interpersonal view of PTSD. Eur J Psychotraumatol. 2016;7 https://doi.org/10.3402/ejpt.v7.29303.
21. Maercker A, Horn AB. A socio-interpersonal perspective on PTSD: the case for environments and interpersonal processes. Clin Psychol Psychother. 2013;20:465–81.
22. Muysewinkel E, Vesentini L, Van Deynse H, et al. Trauma exposure, social support and mental health in the general population in Belgium. Eur J Investig Health Psychol Educ. 2024;14:2047–56.
23. Nalah AB, Ishaya LD. A conceptual overview of deviance and its implication to mental health: a bio psychosocial perspective. Int J Hum Soc Sci Invent.
24. Jankowitz S. The 'Hierarchy of Victims' in Northern Ireland: a framework for critical analysis. Int J Trans Justice. 2018;12:216–36.
25. Gilbert E. Victim compensation for acts of terrorism and the limits of the state. Crit Stud Terror. 2018;11:199–218.
26. Erikson K. Notes on trauma and community. In: Caruth C, editor. Trauma: explorations in memory. Hopkins University Press; 1995.
27. Solomon Z. Oscillating between denial and recognition of PTSD: why are lessons learned and forgotten? J Trauma Stress. 1995;8:271–82.
28. Benjamin J. Acknowledgment of collective trauma in light of dissociation and dehumanization. Psychoanal Perspect. 2011;8:207–14.
29. Danielian J. A century of silence. Am J Psychoanal. 2010;70:245–64.
30. Van Overmeire R. The association between exposure to terrorist attacks and mental health in Belgium. Thesis, Vrije Universiteit Brussel, 2021.
31. Van Overmeire R, Vesentini L, Van Keer R-L, et al. Working experiences of airport employees after a terrorist attack in Belgium: a qualitative study. Int J Disaster Risk Reduct. 2021;64:102515.
32. Friedman-Peleg K, Goodman YC. From posttrauma intervention to immunization of the social body: pragmatics and politics of a resilience program in Israel's periphery. Cult Med Psychiatry. 2010;34:421–42.
33. Durodié B, Wainwright D. Terrorism and post-traumatic stress disorder: a historical review. Lancet Psychiatry. 2019;6:61–71.
34. McLaughlin K. Surviving identity. Routledge, 2013. https://doi.org/10.4324/9780203147665.
35. Letschert R, Ammerlaan K. Compensation and reparation for victims of terrorism. In: Assisting victims of terrorism. Dordrecht: Springer; 2009. p. 215–66.
36. Stene LE, Vuillermoz C, Van OR, et al. Psychosocial care responses to terrorist attacks: a country case study of Norway, France and Belgium. BMC Health Serv Res. 2022;22:390.
37. Fourez G. The legal recognition of victims of terrorism in europe. 2020.
38. Possick C, Shamai M, Sadeh RA. Healing the social self: how parents whose children were killed in terror attacks construct the experience of help. Community Ment Health J. 2014;50:487–96.
39. Joseph J, Jaswal S. Psychosocial framework for understanding psychological distress among survivors of the November 26, 2008 Mumbai terror attack: beyond traumatic experiences and emergency medical care. Prehosp Disaster Med. 2014;29:330–8.
40. Balasinorwala VP, Shah N. Acute stress disorder in victims after terror attacks in Mumbai, India. Br J Psychiatry. 2009;195:462.
41. American Psychiatric Association, editor. *Diagnostic and statistical manual of mental disorders*. 5th ed. American Psychiatric Association; 2013. https://doi.org/10.1176/appi.books.9780890425596.

42. Nixon Rob. Slow violence and the environmentalism of the poor. Harvard University Press; 2013.
43. Rimé B, Páez D, Basabe N, et al. Social sharing of emotion, post-traumatic growth, and emotional climate: Follow-up of Spanish citizen's response to the collective trauma of March 11th terrorist attacks in Madrid. Eur J Soc Psychol. 2010;40:1029–45.
44. Klein O. The lay historian: how ordinary people think about history. In: Cabecinhas R, Abadia L, editors. *Narratives and social memory: theoretical and methodological approaches*. Communication and Society Research Centre; 2013.
45. Charretier L, Eustache F, Laisney M, et al. Narration of a collective traumatic event according to the presence of PTSD and considering the social function. Front Psychiatry. 2024;15 https://doi.org/10.3389/fpsyt.2024.1390470.
46. D'Andrea W, Chiu PH, Casas BR, et al. Linguistic predictors of post-traumatic stress disorder symptoms following 11 September 2001. Appl Cogn Psychol 2012; 26: 316–323.
47. Life For Brussels. Association engagée auprès des victimes d'actes de terrorisme. *Life For Brussels*.
48. V-Europe. Empowering Victims of Terrorism. *V-Europe*, https://v-europe.org/nl_BE. 2026. Accessed 28 February 2026.
49. VRT. En Toen Was Het Stil.
50. Struys B. Minister Verlinden maakt eindelijk werk van 'uniek contactpunt' voor terreur, tien jaar na aanslagen. De Morgen. 2026;
51. Alexander J. Trauma: a social theory. Cambridge: Polity Press; 2012.
52. Schmiedebach H-P. The history of psychotraumatology. In: Trauma Sequelae. Berlin, Heidelberg: Springer; 2022. p. 3–12.
53. Schutt RK. A sociological perspective on disasters. In: Awotona AA, editor. Rebuilding sustainable communities for children and their families after disasters: a global survey. Cambridge Scholars; 2010. p. 458.
54. Miller LM. Controlling disasters: recognising latent goals after Hurricane Katrina. Disasters. 2012;36:122–39.
55. Bullard RD. Differential vulnerabilities: environmental and economic inequality and government response to unnatural disasters. Soc Res Int Q. 2008;75:753–84.
56. Furedi F. The changing meaning of disaster. Area. 39
57. Weisaeth L. The European history of psychotraumatology. J Trauma Stress. 15
58. Mills CW. The sociological imagination. New York: Oxford University PRess; 1959.
59. Horwitz AVV. PTSD: a short history. Johns Hopkins University Press; 2018.
60. Garfield G. Hurricane Katrina: the making of unworthy disaster victims. J Afr Am Stud. 2007;10:55–74.
61. Durkheim E. Suicide. Routledge, 2005. https://doi.org/10.4324/9780203994320.
62. Orjuela C. Navigating labels, seeking recognition for victimhood: diaspora activism after mass-atrocities. Global Netw. 2022;22:166–79.
63. Ursano RJ, Fullerton CS, Weisaeth L, et al. Textbook of disaster psychiatry. Cambridge; 2017.
64. Siampakou N. *Victims of terrorism and reparation applying the* 2005 UN basic principles and guidelines on the right to a remedy and reparation. 2023.
65. Brooks M, O'Brien RO, Livanou M, et al. Collective violence, strengths, and perceived post-traumatic growth: a scoping review. Trauma Violence Abuse. 2025;26:342–55.
66. Li M, Leidner B, Hirschberger G, et al. From threat to challenge: understanding the impact of historical collective trauma on contemporary intergroup conflict. Perspect Psychol Sci. 2023;18:190–209.
67. Erikson K. Everything in its path: destruction of community in the buffalo creek flood. Simon & Schuster; 1976.
68. Thoresen S, Jensen TK, Wentzel-Larsen T, et al. Social support barriers and mental health in terrorist attack survivors. J Affect Disord. 2014;156:187–93.
69. Zalta AK, Tirone V, Orlowska D, et al. Examining moderators of the relationship between social support and self-reported PTSD symptoms: a meta-analysis. Psychol Bull. 2021;147:33–54.

70. Wang Y, Chung MC, Wang N, et al. Social support and posttraumatic stress disorder: a meta-analysis of longitudinal studies. Clin Psychol Rev. 2021;85:101998.
71. Muldoon OT, Haslam SA, Haslam C, et al. The social psychology of responses to trauma: social identity pathways associated with divergent traumatic responses. Eur Rev Soc Psychol. 2019;30:311–48.
72. Harrington R. The railway accident: trains, trauma, and technoloigcal crises in nineteenth-century Britain. In: Traumatic pasts. Cambridge: Cambridge University Press; 2001.
73. Campbell B, Manning J. *The rise of victimhood culture*. Cham: Springer; 2018. https://doi.org/10.1007/978-3-319-70329-9.

# Appendix: Overview of Terrorist Attacks Referred to in this Book

| Year | Country | Short name and characteristics |
|---|---|---|
| 1995 | Japan, Tokyo | Tokyo Sarin attack<br>Religious terrorist attack<br>Sarin in public transport<br>14 people killed |
| 1995 | United States, Oklahoma | Oklahoma City Bombing<br>Anti-government terrorist attack<br>Bombing with truck<br>167 people killed |
| 1998 | Northern Ireland, County Tyrone | Omagh bombing<br>REAL IRA bombing<br>Car bombing<br>29 people killed |
| 1998 | Kenya, Nairobi | Nairobi embassy bombing<br>Islamic terrorist attack<br>Bombings with trucks<br>220 people killed |
| 2001 | United States, New York | 9/11<br>Islamic terrorist attack<br>Four hijacked airplanes used as suicide bombs<br>2977 people killed |
| 2002 | Indonesia, Bali | Bali attacks<br>Islamic terrorist attack<br>Suicide bombs and self-destruct bombs<br>202 people killed |
| 2003 | Turkey, Istanbul | Istanbul attack<br>Islamic terrorist attack<br>Truck bombings<br>28 people killed |

(continued)


R. Van Overmeire, *Terrorism, Mental Health and Aftercare*,
https://doi.org/10.1007/978-3-032-31560-1

(continued)

| Year | Country | Short name and characteristics |
|---|---|---|
| 2004 | Spain, Madrid | Madrid attacks<br>Islamic terrorist attack<br>Train bombings<br>193 people killed |
| 2004 | Russia, Beslan | Beslan attacks<br>Islamic terrorist attack<br>School shootings/hostage taking<br>334 people killed |
| 2005 | England, London | London attacks<br>Islamic terrorist attack<br>Public transport bombings<br>52 people killed |
| 2008 | India, Mumbai | Mumbai attacks<br>Islamic terrorist attack<br>Twelve attacks throughout Mumbai<br>175 people killed |
| 2011 | Norway, Utøya/Oslo attack | Norway/Utøya/Oslo attacks<br>Nationalist terrorist attack<br>Bombings and shooting<br>77 people killed |
| 2013 | United States, Boston | Boston Marathon attacks<br>Islamic terrorist attack<br>Bombings<br>3 people killed |
| 2015 | Tunisia, Tunis | Tunis attack<br>Islamic terrorist attack<br>Shootings<br>21 people killed |
| 2015 | France, Paris | Paris attacks<br>Islamic terrorist attack<br>Bombings and shootings<br>130 people killed |
| 2016 | Belgium, Brussels/Zaventem | Brussels attacks<br>Islamic terrorist attack<br>Suicide bombings<br>32 people killed |
| 2017 | England, Manchester | Manchester attacks<br>Islamic terrorist attack<br>Concert hall bombing<br>22 people killed |
| 2023 | Israel, southern Israel | October 7 attack<br>Islamic terrorist attack<br>Mass attack of terrorist/shootings<br>1195 people killed |

# Index




R. Van Overmeire, *Terrorism, Mental Health and Aftercare*,
https://doi.org/10.1007/978-3-032-31560-1

The manufacturer's authorised representative in the EU is Springer Nature Customer Service Centre GmbH, Europaplatz 3, 69115 Heidelberg, Germany. If you have any concerns regarding our products, please contact ProductSafety@springernature.com

Printed and bound by CPI Group (UK) Ltd, Croydon, CR0 4YY
17/09/2026
02218432-0002